# Understanding Counselling in Primary Care

For Donald Schön

*Authors*

**Marilyn Pietroni** is a BCP registered psychotherapist. She was counsellor and psychotherapist at Marylebone Health Centre from 1992–1998, where she also convened the academic meetings for the multi-professional team, and continues to supervise. She trained as a psychiatric social worker at the London School of Economics and as a psychotherapist at the Tavistock Clinic, where she taught for many years. As Principal Lecturer in Primary Health and Community Care at the University of Westminster, she led the development of postgraduate programmes on inter-professional collaboration.

**Alison Vaspe** is a UKRC registered counsellor who studied music, and worked in publishing before training at Westminster Pastoral Foundation and Birkbeck College, London University. She also has an MA in Psychoanalytic Psychotherapy from the Guild of Psychotherapists/University of Hertfordshire. She works as a counsellor at King's College, London and at the Marylebone Health Centre, where she now leads the team. She is co-editor, with John Lees, of *Clinical Counselling in Further and Higher Education* and is Commissioning Editor of the journal *Psychodynamic Counselling*.

*For Churchill Livingstone:*

*Publishing Manager:* Inta Ozols
*Project Manager:* Derek Robertson

# Understanding Counselling in Primary Care
## Voices from the Inner City

Edited by

## Marilyn Pietroni MA DipSoc CertMH BCPReg
Counsellor and Psychotherapist, Marylebone Health Centre, London;
Principal Lecturer in Primary Health and Community Care,
University of Westminster, London

## Alison Vaspe MMus MA UKRCRegCouns
Counsellor, Marylebone Health Centre, London

Foreword by

## Ellen Noonan AB BA DCP
Head of Counselling Section, Faculty of Continuing Education,
Birkbeck College, London, and Independent Practitioner

Series Editor

## Patrick Pietroni FRCGP MRCP DCH

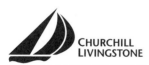
CHURCHILL
LIVINGSTONE

EDINBURGH LONDON NEW YORK PHILADELPHIA ST LOUIS SYDNEY TORONTO 2000

CHURCHILL LIVINGSTONE
An imprint of Harcourt Publishers Limited

© Harcourt Publishers Limited 2000

 is a registered trademark of Harcourt Publishers Limited

The rights of Marilyn Pietroni and Alison Vaspe to be identified as authors of this work have been asserted by them in accordance with the Copyright, Designs and Patents Act 1988

First published 2000

ISBN 0443 05924 1

**British Library Cataloguing in Publication Data**
A catalogue record for this book is available from the British Library

**Library of Congress Cataloging in Publication Data**
A catalog record for this book is available from the Library of Congress

The
publisher's
policy is to use
**paper manufactured
from sustainable forests**

Printed in China

# Contents

# Figures

# Series Editor's Foreword

This is the second book in the series about the work of the Marylebone Health Centre in central London known as the Marylebone Experiment. The first book, *Innovations in Community Care and Primary Health*, addressed the setting up of the centre – the initial research and development work tackled issues in the fields of inner-city deprivation, complementary medicine, counselling, community outreach, patient participation and the nature of organisational life in complex systems.

This book concentrates exclusively on the further development of the counselling service within this interprofessional context. As a result, it becomes possible to describe the service in close up as it evolves. The authors explain how they developed a range of counselling services tailored to the known patterns of patient need. They also discuss how they maximised the use of their scarce resources, reflecting their recognition of the importance of the context of the counselling service, as well as its content and nature. These innovations also provided recently qualified counsellors and psychotherapists with an opportunity to work under supervision in the somewhat pressured and difficult environment of the health centre, whilst increasing the range of counselling approaches available to the patients. Finally, using the voices of the patients themselves, the authors take the reader through the minefield of interacting perspectives that surround and make up the counselling work itself.

One of the stages en route is the counsellors' contribution to increasing rigour in the practice in relation to the terminology used in the multi-professional team. Using a reflective practice approach, and not flinching from the sometimes painful discoveries of unrecognised differences that this exposes, the authors review an important investigation into the much used and abused term of 'containment' in the multi-professional team. Here, the fragile links between theory and practice are examined, and conflicts in meaning are revealed, before a new common language can be established.

A final word about this book. It will not go without notice that one of the authors happens also to be my wife! We have worked together in this field, on and off, for about the last fifteen years. Together, we developed the six-stage stress management programme in Cincinnati, from which the Marylebone model originated before it was further developed by the health centre team in association with the University of Westminster. The chemistry of collaboration is often invisible but this book goes some way to revealing its complexity and depth.

Future books in the series will concentrate on specific features of the Marylebone experiment: the work of the complementary therapists and on the community outreach unit.

Patrick Pietroni

# Foreword

Counselling in general practice is coming of age as a specialist brand of counselling in the UK. Like its sibling branches in, say, education and the workplace, it has had to argue first for its existence and then has had to find a way to manage the flood of unpredictable demand on underresourced services. The arguments of justification are very similar – that counselling is indirectly cost effective, that 'talking through' a problem is preferable to symptomatic relief through mechanical, chemical, bureaucratic or draconian means and is likely to be a longer lasting solution. And the operational problems are also similar – how to manage growing waiting lists and the frustrating ambivalence of clients who 'waste' precious counsellor time by not attending; how to manage the counsellor's attachment to their clients and to the notion of long-term work that finishes when the job is done (mutual termination versus the arbitrary contract of a preset number of sessions); how to provide a low cost (free to clients) service which is necessarily staffed by expensive (i.e. highly trained) professionals who require decent accommodation and support as part of their occupational equipment. The similarities can feel dispiriting because it seems that one branch does not learn from the experience of another and ends up working out resolutions from scratch. This may be because it is hard to imagine that the settings share anything – the kinds of problems met in the classroom, the office, the GP's surgery are surely very different and the outcomes surely very specific to the requirements or desires of the referrers. It may also be because counselling has only just begun to develop a research and publish mentality, so knowledge about the establishment and running of a service remains quite local and private. Public sharing at conferences and meetings too often takes the form of exasperation with the institutions which house the services in an inverted rivalry about who is hardest done by The Management. Pending audit processes raise sighs of resentment or frisson of panic.

This book may be a break-through in this respect. As it chronicles the history of the development of one particular service, it has some of the qualities of a fly-on-the-wall documentary and of a do-it-yourself manual. It is, of course, a very particular service, predicated on a holistic approach to medicine in which the response to the problems of patients is based on taking the whole of the person into account, not just the ailing part. The success of this integrated multi-functional, inter-professional approach lies in exploring the boundaries and barriers between conventional and complementary medicine, between psychological and physical remedies. A cluster of chapters record the minutiae of a counsellor's day or year in the practice. It shows how they juggle the vicissitudes of getting to work, the administrative chores that make up the infrastructure of the service and its links with the health centre as a whole, the fostering of professional relationships and professional ideas, and giving undistracted attention to their clients in the sessions and through supervision. The mechanics of the work are presented in some detail: the service menu, the referral process, the communication signals, the schedule of meetings, and so on. All these activities and processes are regarded as every bit as important as the client session itself to the success of the care, and cure, of the individual patient within the practice. The chapter on containment powerfully demonstrates how differences which threaten to disrupt the collaboration can be tackled patiently in a way that marshals professional resource rather than professional rivalry, and the whole enterprise is infused with an understated firmness about the arrangements and a security of belief in them that ensures that they are adhered to. Such serious and equitable attention to the processes and relationships also automatically attends to questions about efficiency, effectiveness, and cost so that an audit poses little threat. It is heartening to read this account which embraces rather than grudges and defends against scrutiny.

The chapter on containment is pivotal to the work described here. Not only does it track the working through of differences of definition and consequent action of this core concept, but it also is a live example of reflective practice as defined by Schön, who is the invisible mentor in the work. Schön stresses the necessity of linking the elegant 'high ground' of intellectual understanding with the murky 'swamp' of everyday practice. The unpredictable and emotional force that sweeps into the room with every patient-client can, as every counsellor knows, unseat the mind with disconcerting ease, which makes a nice clean academic seminar discussion all the more attractive in defence against helplessness. Finding the unknowable uniqueness of each encounter, drawing on thought and feeling in a way that permits each to enrich the other, is what all counsellors strive for. This is curiously paralleled in the review of literature on counselling in general practice. It is inconclusive; there are so many factors, so little typicality that it is hard to generalize, but there is something to be learned from everything.

The third section of the book on practice addresses the subtitle 'Voices from the Inner City'. The familiar link between the stress of urban life and physical illness will prepare the reader for some of the content of these six selected cases, but they nonetheless come as quite a shock as the severity of the problems, and the way that those extensively disable the lives of the sufferers, unfold in the accounts. These counsellors are dealing with agonized grief, paralysing depression, unbearable anxiety, terror and torture. I think it is true to say that these problems could turn up in any setting, which argues again for my proposition that different branches of counselling can and should be learning from each other, but the quality that sets this work apart is that everyone in and around the health centre pulls together and makes use of the skills and perceptions of the others. The GP makes the referral, having already given the patient considerable attention; the receptionists contribute from their front-line position; the supervisor lends support and insight; the practice nurse is also part of the mesh of the net which provides safety and transformation. Most of these case studies focus on professional relationships within the practice, but there are other vignettes in the book which involve the providers of complementary medicine and the social agencies in the neighbourhood in the same way. The accounts also indicate how the carefully devised service menu provides a reliable structure for managing the pace of work with each client. Each account concludes with a reflection on the work in terms of the values and principles of the service and on the impact of postmodern inner city pressures on particular groups of vulnerable people.

The dialogue between inner and outer continues throughout the book. The counselling relationship is described as a 'rare and special opportunity for patients to have that "still point" in the [busy] practice when they can think and talk within a clear time/space,' and for this it is to be valued not only by patients but by all professionals and even society at large. It does seem, however, that the work described here also allows the professionals a still point where they can voice their anxieties about their work and have those heard, contained and worked with. More than that, it allows people a place to make use of the often unspoken thoughts that we all have and find privately interesting but tend to squander because there is seldom a place to say them. The receptionist who notices that a patient is invisible to her is perhaps a small detail, but in context it gains significance which sheds light on the patient, helps the counsellor, and involves the receptionist in the team. Focussing on the tiny detail while seeing it as a reflection of the widest social force, dealing with unconscious relationships in the complex net of collaborative activities, balancing the needs of the individual with the needs of the market are some aspects of the dialogue, but of course it is the dialogue itself which has made the work of the centre so impressive. Putting it all into words for others to read is a generous act on the part of the authors. Everyone reading from here will certainly be stimulated and educated by these voices of experience.

Ellen Noonan

# Acknowledgements

We wish to acknowledge the contributions of the patients and the multi-professional team and community networks at Marylebone Health Centre without whom the book could not have been written. Similarly our families, notably Patrick Pietroni, Peter Vaspe, colleagues especially Romayne Jesty and Anne Kilcoyne, and the editorial team at Churchill Livingstone, Valerie Dearing and Inta Ozols, have tolerated and supported us through the joy and pain of writing and producing this book. Thanks are also due to the University of Westminster who funded part of Marilyn Pietroni's time. For any errors of fact or misinterpretations of material however, the authors alone are responsible.

# Introduction

Where past and future are gathered. Neither movement from nor towards,
Neither descent nor decline. Except for the point, the still point,
There would be no dance, and there is only the dance.

T.S.Eliot, *The Four Quartets*

Counselling can provide one of the 'still points' where thinking can take place in general practice. The fifty minute or half-hour counselling session in which there is time to listen, to think and to try to understand can seem like a luxury in a setting where ten minute sessions with the GP and fifteen patients per two hour surgery are the norm. However sometimes what confronts the counsellor in an inner city practice in terms of gathering 'past and future' together is profoundly disturbing: refugees who have been tortured, marriages that have been fractured, young people adrift and in turmoil, elders and very sick people living out the shreds of their life alone. For these people the counsellor is only one point of contact in a maze of others.

We aim to show the activity of counselling in inner city general practice as it happens in one practice, rather than to teach about it in general. We try to give a living picture of the realities through the words and thoughts of those who make up the service: the patients, the GPs, the receptionists, the practice nurses, the counsellors and, because this is a book about the Marylebone Health Centre, the complementary therapy team. The first book on the work of the health centre was published in this Churchill Livingstone series as *Innovations in community care and primary health: the Marylebone experiment* (Pietroni & Pietroni 1996).

In Donald Schön's words, we are concerned with 'the swamp' of frontline work in the inner city where 'real-world problems do not come well-formed' but 'rather tend to present themselves as messy, indeterminate,problematic situations' (1992, p.53). Here things do not always go according to plan, and reflection on the surprises and dilemmas of practice contribute to modifications of both theory and technique in the process of developing an informed pragmatism. General practitioners have to be pragmatic. They have to manage 'six minutes for the patient' (Balint & Norell 1973), and cope several times a day with the last minute 'while I'm here, doctor' (Elder & Samuel 1987). We believe that counsellors need to develop pragmatism to work effectively in this setting with GPs and interprofessionally in the team. The counselling service we describe has been developed in this spirit and forms part of the overall clinical services at Marylebone Health Centre in Central London.

The first part of the book is about the inner city context of counselling at Marylebone Health Centre, and sets the scene for what follows. General practice has been described by Wiener as like a souk or bazaar (1996), and certainly for any counsellor who has not worked in the setting before, this graphic description captures well the exotic mix and unexpected rhythms of the work. We begin with an account of each of our working days: Marilyn Pietroni's first day in 1993 when there was only one counsellor at the practice, and one of Alison Vaspe's recent days after a counselling team of three has been established and a menu of varied counselling services developed.

This first joint chapter shows how we managed our joint authorship. We write and work differently, and have different backgrounds and levels of experience, a picture which is common in general practice counselling. Early on in our collaboration we decided to allow our differences free rein, with one of us taking lead responsibility for writing each chapter, whilst exchanging drafts for feedback as work progressed.

Chapter 2 is about the inner city community of Marylebone and describes how Marylebone Health Centre developed a flexible, inter-professional service to meet the varied needs that exist. The Marylebone Model of Primary Health Care is illustrated by the 'Flower Diagram' (Fig. 2.1 p.30) which acts as a frame for the inter-professional approach and shows how the counselling service fits into the whole. Each part of the whole is illustrated by a vignette: a small example that shows the service at work in all its different aspects. The chapter also shows how complex the setting of general practice is, with its part-timers and full-timers, the on-call system, and the range of adjacent community health agencies and professions that make up the extended primary care team. The chapter therefore also describes how communication structures are set in place to hold this complex system of activities together through a regular programme of meetings and academic development, in records and on a day-by-day basis.

The next two chapters describe the way that the counselling service at Marylebone Health Centre has developed and now works. The service is part of the general practice system and does not function independently in the way that, for example, some private or independent counselling services do. The counsellors at Marylebone work individually and are each quite different but they are also team players who have chosen to adapt their practice to suit the needs of the patients and the nature of the practice environment, at the same time as influencing that environment in specific ways. These two chapters describe how they have done so.

The fifth chapter gives a profile of one year's work in the counselling service at Marylebone Health Centre. Each year the practice staff write an annual report based on audit data which is available on request from the practice manager. In it the work of each of the units in the multi-professional team is analyzed and described. The pattern of the counselling service over a five year period is fairly stable, so the picture of any one year gives a good picture of the overall demands on and activities of the service. This chapter concludes Part 1.

Part 2, 'Working debates', tackles the conceptual and evidence-base for the work but in the same pragmatic spirit. In Chapter 6, key issues in the expanding literature are addressed. Much important work has gone to print recently (notably Wiener & Sher 1998, Burton 1998 and Lees 1999), so this chapter is like a snapshot at one point in time, drawing out some of the key issues but inevitably partial. The rapidly changing context of national health and social care policy is signalled and we take it very seriously. However, the policy environment has not been addressed in detail. Not only are there many excellent books on the subject which accomplish this task with considerable expertise, for example, *Going inter-professional* edited by Audrey Leathard (1996), but also, at the time of writing, a new Labour government was in the midst of recasting the massive changes that had taken place under the Conservative administration since 1990.

Research priorities tend mostly to be determined by government policy. During the last ten years market forces have shaped the agenda in health and social care following major legislative change in the late eighties and early nineties. Much of the existing literature on counselling in general practice inevitably, therefore, tends to bring to the foreground issues of efficiency, economy and effectiveness in response to those frequently asked questions: Do counsellors maximize the use of scarce resources? Does counselling work? Is it value for money? These are important questions which need answers, but they can often be approached in the literature without an accompanying picture of the complexity of both the setting and the work.

Such a picture needs to give a different emphasis to the questions and requires descriptions as well as analysis. What do counsellors actually do in general practice? How do they fit into the team? What do patients bring to them? What are their particular dilemmas? How do they relate to resource constraints? As counsellors at Marylebone Health Centre, we are as much a part of the 'care culture' of general practice in the inner city as we are of the 'cure culture'. Outcome studies will therefore need to concentrate primarily on patient satisfaction. Clinically significant change measures collected throughout counselling rather than the traditional before and after studies are, however, now recommended in the literature (Burton 1998). The intrusiveness of information gathering for such studies on very brief work of the kind with which we are mainly concerned has to be borne in mind. We do indicate certain outcome areas where money has been saved by the preventive aspects of counselling at Marylebone, through reduced prescription charges and GP attendance rates, but more research in this area is needed. On the whole, the book we have written here is in a different vein. Our aim has been to contribute to the literature in a different way, and from a reflective practice point of view, by telling the first-hand story of one counselling service in one general practice at work.

Chapter 7, 'Reflective practice and the post modern context', provides a rationale for the pragmatic approach to counselling in general practice taken at Marylebone Health Centre, and for the 'local story' approach that we have taken in this book. In Chapter 8, 'Theory in use: perspectives on containment', a conceptual building block which is much used in counselling and in other forms of therapeutic practice is examined, first abstractly and then drawing on the fruits of inter-professional debate from the Academic Meetings at Marylebone Health Centre. The term containment was much used in the team discussions at the practice, so for one year the monthly academic meetings were used to explore and refine its meaning; in other words to 'ground' the theory. Perhaps not surprisingly, it was discovered that different members of the multi-professional team were using the term quite differently. These different 'meanings in use' were therefore an invisible barrier in team communication which undermined inter-professional collaboration and patient care. In the course of the year, the team rebuilt the term from scratch into three simpler shared meanings to which everyone could subscribe. These meanings were defined in everyday rather than professional language to ensure accessibility and commonality and to reduce mystification between the professions. This process of unscrambling misunderstandings and creating new meanings also enabled the different professions in the team to begin to understand each other's worlds and to move from a *multi-professional* approach, where professions simply work alongside each other, to an *inter-professional* approach where collaboration takes place based on a genuine understanding of differences.

Part 3 'Inside counselling in the inner city', moves the counselling service into close-up. We have selected a series of typical stories of what happened in and around six episodes of counselling, using as far as possible the words of those involved: the patients, the counsellors, the GPs, the practice nurses, the receptionists and those in other agencies where relevant. The material for the stories was gathered from process recordings of sessions, from semi-structured interviews and from records. To give the sense of work which is unfolding, and often unclear and uncertain, we have used the actual words of those involved, including speech discontinuities. As these stories are offered raw, with little commentary, we have inserted occasional information boxes that provide emphasis or information, identify key dilemmas or note general learning points. The stories sometimes include contradictions and ambiguities because these were present as a living feature of the situation or the work that took place. To eradicate them would have presented a smoother finish, but would have distorted the real nature of the work. Where work is continuing, we have sought and been given consent by the patients concerned to publish their stories in their own words. We have in all stories changed key facts to protect confidentiality.

Part 4, 'The global city', offers by way of a postscript some concluding thoughts about the need for quiet yet accurate listening to the voices from the inner city. As Eliot (1944) puts it, 'Except for the point, the still point/There would be no dance, and there is only the dance.' Thus improvisation and routine are both needed to meet the often turbulent inner worlds of patients who live in the inner city and present in a multi-professional general practice setting, amidst what Balint called 'the harmonious interpenetrating mix-up' of environment and individual (Balint 1968 p.72).

## Note on terminology

Throughout this book the terms counsellor and psychotherapist are used interchangeably, following the example of Launer (1994) and because the research on and activity of brief psychotherapy is highly relevant to our subject. Counsellors have a clear system of regulation and accreditation through the British Association of Counselling (BAC) and are usually trained in brief work. The world of psychotherapy is divided between the United Kingdom Confederation of Psychotherapists (UKCP) and the British Confederation of Psychotherapists (BCP). The literature on counselling in general practice is however of one view: that psychotherapists and counsellors, whatever their training or persuasion, need to adapt their practice to the different needs and rhythms of the setting and must be trained and experienced in very brief work.

# PART 1

# Context: counselling at Marylebone Health Centre

# Then and now: two days in the life of counselling in general practice

*Marilyn Pietroni\* and Alison Vaspe*

The despoliation of our cities concerns me not just as a Londoner but as a doctor because it generates a great deal of ill-health, depression and family disruption [...] People are a city, populations allowed some stability to grow and work and educate themselves.

David Widgery, *Some lives*

## SYNOPSIS

Inner city general practice can be quite a shock for counsellors or psychotherapists who are unfamiliar with the setting.

Here, Marilyn Pietroni writes about her first day's work in general practice in 1992. The story she tells is one of high emotional impact resulting from the range of raw, and sometimes shocking, problems brought by people who are struggling with their lives in the inner city.

By 1998 Alison Vaspe has been at the practice several years, as part of the now developed counselling team, and has recently taken over management of new referrals and the waiting list. A varied Menu of Counselling Services is now well established and is described in more detail in Chapter 3.

Alison's story provides an insight into how carefully the counsellor manages herself and her resources in what is by now a semi-structured system. It shows how even the 10-minute breaks between patients are made productive in terms of liaison and small management tasks as well as finding 'the still point' for thinking and digesting the impact of the counselling work itself.

The two stories aim to give a sense of development over a six year period from a lone counsellor working in a new setting, to being a member of a counselling team working to a shared policy which relates limited resources to a wide variety of clinical needs.

---

\*Marilyn Pietroni's contribution to this chapter is based on a workshop presentation at the MIND Conference, London, 1994 subsequently published in *Psychodynamic Counselling* 3 July 1995. Volume 1 Number 3.

## THEN (1992)

*Marilyn Pietroni*

It was with some trepidation that I approached my first day's counselling in general practice. My past experience of counselling had been over a number of years in social work, and in a university and a mental health clinic, mainly with adults but also in the past with young people and their families. I was also an experienced adult psychotherapist and had worked in several hospital settings, both general and psychiatric, but never in general practice. I was curious about this front line generalist setting, about the kinds of problems that people might bring, and about the rush of referrals that had occurred prior to my arrival. I also wondered how a counsellor would be related to by the multi-professional staff team of the health centre. My first day's experience had a profound effect on me.

The receptionists were the first point of contact on arrival in the practice and I was struck by their combination of warmth and firmness with both staff and patients. Somehow they managed to answer the incessantly ringing telephone, handle the front desk and appointments book, 'pull' the notes for all the surgeries and clinical appointments of the day, and pass the time of day with whoever was passing. As I observed them carry out these tasks, I felt this strangely ordered chaos was my first lesson about working in general practice. Mistakes were addressed in a matter-of-fact way, appointments were rescheduled if necessary, limits were set, people in trouble were given kindly attention, those who were too demanding were put in their place. Sometimes the receptionists (all women) seemed at risk from upset or disturbed patients who could not get what they wanted. Sometimes there were just not enough of them to do all that there was to do.

As this disciplined chaos took place in front of my eyes, I reflected more on what went on behind the consulting room doors. Would I be able to cope? I had, as part of my induction, sat in on several GP surgeries and had wondered how GPs developed the capacity to see and respond to such a wide variety of patients and problems in such a short time. I had also been shocked that people came to their doctor with some very minor ailments such as coughs and colds, or routine aches and pains. Would this trivialization be reflected in the counselling referrals also?

## The built environment

The health centre is located in the crypt of a church on a busy main road and the crypt space is divided into five: art exhibitions, a small chapel open to the public, a cafe open until tea-time daily, a healing and counselling service run by the church (and often confused with our own) and the health centre itself. Access from the street is by a spiral staircase or by lift.

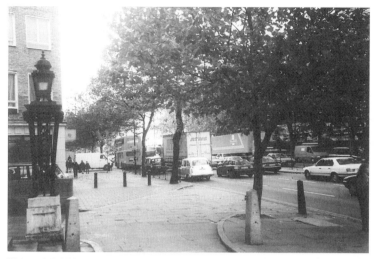

**Figure 1.1**  Marylebone Road

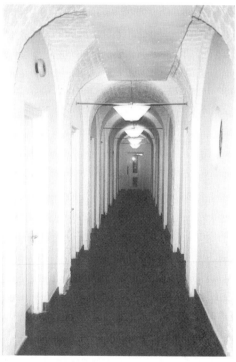

**Figure 1.2**  The counselling room corridor

Architecturally simple and beautiful, the crypt seems at first to offer an atmosphere of tranquillity away from the bustle of the Marylebone Road. As a workspace, however, there is a problem with air circulation and it is difficult to adjust to the lack of fresh air and daylight (Figs 1.1 & 1.2).

The counselling room I had been given was simple: whitewashed with a beautiful arched ceiling but windowless, stuffy and without a telephone or intercom. A panic button was provided for use in emergency. The room was two corridors away from the health centre reception and I found myself uncertain about how to manage this arrangement logistically if a patient was late. To wait in reception or to wait in the consulting room? I did not want to hover awkwardly so I opted for the latter, with patients knocking on the consulting room door before entering.

## Time and patterns of work

I was only too aware of the need for counselling in general practice and of the time pressures posed by insufficient resources. I began by working two half days a week. Each half-day session was $3\frac{1}{2}$ hours, and I decided to offer two 30-minute sessions each half day to increase access. This would mean four 50-minute and four half-hour sessions per week. I was familiar with half-hour sessions from my days in the psychiatric outpatients department and from Hill End Adolescent Unit. I knew 'short' sessions were both possible and potentially useful (Bruggen, Byng-Hall & Pitt Aitken 1973), I was aware that Balint had defined half an hour as a 'long' GP session (1964), I felt I was experienced enough to assess and respond carefully. I had set up a simple GP referral form that told me a little about the GP's view of the presenting problem, whether or not there was a psychiatric history or the patient had received counselling or psychotherapy in the past, and whether any other workers in the health centre or its local inter-agency network were in any way involved.

## The first referrals

The following four referrals made up my first afternoon's work.

• First patient: A young mother in her mid-30s with panic attacks that had worsened and now occurred while she was in the park with her 4-year-old son as well as at work. Her husband was a driver, she a secretary. She had no previous therapy or psychiatric history. She was seen for 30 minutes and offered brief work of up to six half-hour sessions (the forerunner of what was later known as Service E (see page 51)).

• Second patient: A schoolteacher, male, also mid-30s, with depression and general lack of motivation for life, threatened with redundancy. The GP felt he needed time to look at his problems in greater depth. He too was seen for thirty minutes for the first session only and then offered brief work of six fifty minute sessions on a weekly basis (forerunner of Service B).

• Third patient: A young Arab man, married but separated, just out of hospital after a serious suicide attempt (drinking bleach and an overdose of paracetamol). He was waiting for a follow-up psychiatric appointment. His recent history showed bouts of depression and problems with visa status and accommodation. He was seen for fifty minutes and offered very brief work of up to four weekly sessions pending his hospital appointment (forerunner of Services A and D)

• Fourth patient: A single woman in her 40s wanting to talk to someone about a serious trauma as a teenager which she had never previously discussed. There was no previous psychiatric history. She was seen for fifty minutes and offered brief work with fifty minute sessions on a weekly basis (forerunner of Service B).

## Impact of the first referrals

Although these referrals individually did not go beyond my expectations in terms of range of presenting problems, seriousness of disturbance and range of social class and situation, collectively they did. I could feel in no uncertain terms the impact of *general* practice: the complex switches from one problem to another without respite in between, the dramatically different needs of the patients and expectations from the referrers. I began already to regret my decision to offer half-hour sessions to the first and second referrals.

Only one of the GPs had gone out of their way to discuss the referral personally with me and I became aware of what an enormous difference that made to me but felt pessimistic about introducing such discussions for every referral. That discussion made me aware of just how much a GP can understand from a 5–10 minute consultation. With the other three patients, seeing them for the first time felt like a step into the unknown, in spite of the pre-figuring referral.

Bearing the label of counsellor also made me feel accessible and ordinary in a useful kind of way, but at the same time exposed and uncertain. There was no doubt that this label conferred less status and mystique than the label of psychotherapist with which I was more familiar and I wondered how I would manage that change.

What follows is a summary of the counselling work undertaken with the third and fourth patients because the stories that unfold, and the use of the counselling space and the person of the counsellor, is so different for each that it conveys a good picture of the contrasts of counselling in general practice. Key facts and details have been changed to protect anonymity.

### Third patient

As I collected this patient from the waiting room, I became aware of his formality and courtesy at the same time as a huge weight of some kind, expressed through his haunted eyes and gaunt cheeks, that contrasted with his proud, upright bearing. Although he was wearing Western dress, I wondered how he would feel about seeing a woman and a non-Moslem. He would know that I already knew his history and why he had come. The GP who referred him was male.

I began by telling him how long the session would be and that we could arrange further sessions after today if he wanted and it seemed appropriate. Then I asked what had brought him. He looked first at me and then at the floor and without hesitation or elaboration told the horrific story of his marriage. After a childhood of brutality from a series of stepmothers in his home country, he came to England to study. Because he was fiercely ambitious, single-minded (and very bright) he did well and got a first-class degree. He was contracted to return home to work, but he met and was 'actively' pursued by a woman who ran her own business. She was not a Moslem but neither was he devout, he 'only followed the morality' and the conventions of clean-living and clean-speaking. In a short time he married her and for the first time in his life he had felt happy. He gave up his post-graduate studies and went into the business to help his wife.

All went well for about six months and then they ran into financial problems as the business began to fail. He worked harder and harder but his wife began taking long lunch hours and then going out alone in the evening, something she had never done before. He remonstrated with her but she ridiculed him and taunted him about his ideas. He sometimes felt he wanted to hit her and felt guilty and ashamed at having such a thought because, having been beaten himself, he had made a vow to live a non-violent life. He felt helpless and hurt and she just went on leaving him alone and treating him with contempt. She began to dress provocatively and to spend money that they did not have. Then she left him altogether and, for some reason which he still did not understand, took his passport with her and disappeared 'abroad'. He now felt lonely, stateless and terrified, particularly of the annual immigration interview which was coming up shortly. Most of all he felt humiliated as a man. It was unthinkable in his own country that a man would be left and humiliated in this way by a woman.

I had said nothing as he told his story. Time had run on and there were only about fifteen minutes of the session left. He still had not mentioned being in hospital or his suicide attempt and I knew he had no psychiatric support. It was more hazardous to let him go without referring to it, so I said, 'And then you decided to put an end to it all.' 'I tried,' he said, 'but they found me. Now I have that shame too. Now I can never go back. I am not a man any more.' Then he made a movement with both arms, lifting them above his head. As he did so, he lifted his hair revealing that under a wig he was quite bald.

'This is why I am not a man any more,' he said. I sat feeling physically stunned and profoundly moved. Although dramatic, he had told his story with dignity and simplicity and I felt moved by his courage. His hair had fallen out during the time that he was married and his wife had suggested the wig. For that she had never taunted him and he was grateful as for him it was the biggest burden of all.

I asked if he would like to come back again and talk some more and he said he would. He came for a further four sessions before the hospital caught up with him and offered him a psychiatric referral with the likelihood of psychotherapy, which he decided to take up. So one day he just stopped coming to his sessions. It seemed right that he should take up the referral but it made an abrupt ending. He seemed able to use me to get through that isolated phase when he returned home from hospital. In the last session he had recovered some vitality, and the sexuality and intimacy in the transference were palpable. I made no transference interpretations, however, except in relation to my being a woman and a non-Moslem and, when he was talking about his losses, to the fact that as the sessions would be limited I too, would be leaving him soon. In relation to the former he said, 'You are a professional', in a fairly assertive way and in relation to the latter he shrugged somewhat cynically as if to say, 'Well what else can one expect?'

### Fourth patient

This forty two-year-old woman was referred by her GP, who wrote that she had suffered a 'serious trauma' in her teens and thought she 'might be ready to talk about it now'. There was no indication of what the trauma might be although I found myself wondering before seeing her if it might be some form of abuse. I tried to clear my mind and be ready simply to listen and think, but found this difficult to do after seeing three new patients consecutively already that afternoon. I wished that I could find some way to hold time still so I could recover a more reflective state of mind and yet still not be late.

Here the architectural form of the arched corridor, the simple white decor of the crypt and the walk to the waiting room came to my rescue. Was there some way to plan the sequence of seeing patients in general practice, I wondered? All that training and experience I had had, where was it now? I felt knocked sideways by the last patient with little warning that the effect would be so profound. Now what was ahead? By the time I picked up the fourth patient from the waiting room it seemed a hundred thoughts had passed through my mind in an undigested way. They would have to be put 'on hold' for at least another hour, time to see this patient, think about her and then more fully meet up with myself again.

As I met her I thought how young she looked for someone of her age, positively girlish as, with a slightly awkward outstretched hand, she greeted me and smiled. Seeing her readiness concentrated my attention on the moment and on her. I walked more slowly and deliberately to the room this time and as I closed the door and we each sat down I felt ready to hear her story. I began as before and also explained that her doctor had said she wanted to talk, perhaps, among other things, about something that happened a long time ago. She looked at the floor and laughed a slightly sideways ironic laugh that was to become very familiar over the next few months. It almost seemed to say dismissively, 'How extraordinary to bother to say that about me.' Immediately afterwards though, and as I was to discover, also in a characteristically measured way, she said very slowly, 'Yes, I did actually say that, didn't I?' I was by this time feeling I had plunged in on what was inevitably a big topic, when I should have given her the chance to start more at her own pace.

After my slightly awkward beginning and her response, I waited and so did she. The awkwardness seemed to dissolve. I watched her thinking and then in a very swift and matter-of-fact way she gave me some details about herself that 'I might want to know': her age, her job, where she lived, summed up with a comment something like 'not much to tell', again the irony undercutting both herself and any interest that might be shown by me.

Mindful of my earlier blunder, I waited again for a rather longer time. She seemed to be building up to saying something else, something more important. Her concentration was intense and communicated itself. She gave me the clear feeling that time was rare and precious to her and that she knew how to use it. I must wait and trust her. So I did. I stopped worrying about time as she seemed to have such a good handle on it. 'People tell me I am very precise,' again with that smile, 'I will try to be as we don't have long and I don't want to waste your time.' The following story is changed to protect confidentiality but the substance is true.

When she was a teenager, her parents' marriage broke up over several years. She lived with her mother who had lived in a state of breakdown in and out of hospital during that time. One day, when returning at the weekend from a visit to her father, she found her mother dead in the bathroom having cut her own throat with a carving knife. No-one else was in so she left the house and returned to her father's place and the police were called. She had not talked it over since with anyone in the family and only one close friend knew about it. She thought she felt ready at long last to look back.

For the first time, she looked at me face to face to see how I had taken her story. There was no sense of satisfaction at having opened the door on her story, only what seemed like a kind of worried curiosity at what it might have done to me. 'I'm not sure I'm going to be able to do this,' she said. I replied, 'And you're not sure I'm going to be able to bear it either, are you?' 'No,' she said and stared rather miserably at the floor. I said I would see her again and we could talk some more if she wanted to make another appointment. She nodded.

Working with this patient was a remarkable experience. In over twenty years of practice as a psychotherapist and of supervising others, I have rarely encountered such measured concentration on the essentials. She had a kind of austere self-containment in which her anguish and outrage were at first 'managed', then felt, but not overwhelmingly so. Her wry humour and her intelligent capacity for survival and self-protection had carried her through. She was a mistress of understatement. She did not dramatize any of what she said but made it clear that she needed a particular quality of attention, of listening and of clarity that would do justice to her own internal discipline. One day I talked to her about how tough that discipline was, how little respite there was, how little time for more ordinary life to enter in. This was after about six or seven sessions and we were set to go on for about ten. She grinned and said she had a surprise to tell me – she had booked a long trip overseas and she had fixed up some driving lessons for her return.

In the previous weeks this patient had worked hard and systematically. In some it could have felt contrived to go for the first time to visit her mother's grave, to face the relatives who had kept her away from the funeral because she 'would be too upset' and who had concealed information from her. In this patient, these tasks, set by herself in her own way, were carried out with dignity and without inflicting her own wounds and anger on others. She started a journal (her idea not mine), using it sparingly but to most effect when the work came to an end as a means of self-reflection. In the last session also, she brought back a small flag of friendship from her trip and left it with me saying, 'I know parting gifts are not allowed.' I gave her the details of the colleague she would see privately for a further ten sessions, with money she had managed to save.

Taking a long-term view, some might argue that this patient somewhat controlled the counselling space and time and even the counsellor, me. There is a real technical issue of how to work with well-established defences in short-term work in the setting of general practice. Perhaps I had been caught in the kind of ordered respect that she demanded from people but which created an emotional distance, leaving her enisled with her pain and with the drawbridge drawn up? I do not think so.

She, like the previous patient, was in touch with extreme pain and considerable anger, and was containing that emotion, if somewhat perilously, and knew how, when and where to make use of me, the counsellor, even though I felt deeply unsure myself. I have since come to regard such psychic certainty and sureness of touch, despite the patients' quite different uses of me, as characteristic of counselling in general practice when it goes well.

That first day, all patients arrived, something I now know to be unusual. Counselling in general practice has a rhythm. These opening experiences were just the beginning.

## Postscript

I kept the two thirty minute sessions going for about the first three months, but found it was too difficult at that time because I had a lot of new learning to do. I believe, however, that it was right to try. Some year and a half later, I was able to reinstate those sessions and use them well. I had by then developed a more precise sense of how to do so: for follow-ups, for crises and for those severely mentally ill people who can use counselling as long as it is carefully bounded, regular but infrequent and focused (a kind of psychiatric outpatients' service of the listening variety). By using the short sessions in this way, the waiting list was completely cleared except at difficult times of the year, such as Christmas and New Year. Later, we developed the half-hour sessions into an explicit service listed on the Patient Counselling Self-Request Form as Service E. These services are described in detail in Chapter 3.

## NOW (1998)

*Alison Vaspe*

At the time of writing, I have been working at the health centre for four years. I go in on Wednesday mornings and am employed for one session a week, or three and a half hours. This tends to extend itself either side, which is a hazard of such condensed employment but common, I know, for counsellors in general practice. However, I am aware that all the team find themselves putting in extra time – the GPs, receptionists, practice nurses, counsellors and complementary therapists. It's not a good thing but it's not just me.

I started at the health centre as a voluntary counsellor but have now been paid for three years. I achieved my BAC (British Association of Counsellors) accreditation, partly as a result of my first supervised year at the practice as part of the Counsellor Volunteer and Supervision scheme (described in Chapter 4), and decided to stay on afterwards. I also work with medical and dental students at a South London hospital. I seem to have entered into the medical world in a big way. This sometimes seems strange, for someone who studied music and then worked in publishing, moving from music books to fiction and literary non-fiction, to women writing autobiography. In some way, though, it doesn't feel strange but more like a necessary experience of something important and different. There is a connection which I'm becoming more aware of. But it is something to do with the connection between hearing and feeling music and being alert to one's body as well as one's mind. John Berger made me realize this when he wrote in his novel *Once in Europa*: 'What's so surprising about music is that it comes from the outside. It feels as if it comes from the inside' (Berger 1989).

The common theme of medicine in the hospital and general practice settings does not make working in the two places a very similar experience. The tight discipline of general practice and the rather confined nature of the setting are in contrast to the long hospital corridors and the much greater length of time I spend there. The hospital is also a much more anonymous place. I have worked there for over three years now and am still coming upon new places and new groups of people. The danger in hospitals is of being lost in it all, and a fear is of being forgotten – like the stories of patients left on trolleys, unattended. In general practice, if you are in, you are in. I have an image in my mind here of seeing one of our GPs talking to a distressed patient in the waiting area that lies between the health centre itself and the counselling rooms at the other end of the crypt.

Sometimes, for a counsellor, the GPs are a hard act to follow, but I have grown increasingly interested in how patients who request counselling are often exploring, however tentatively, a different way of thinking about the aches and pains and sometimes the agonies of living in the inner city: a way of feeling that can come out of the body and find some expression in words as they pass between patient and counsellor.

Wednesday is the day when I am at both the general practice and the hospital. I start fairly early by travelling from my home to Baker Street, about an hour and a half's journey. In the middle of the day I cross London again from north to south on my way to the hospital. The travelling makes for an anxious time, worrying about public transport and how many minutes it will allow me before my first booked appointment of the morning or the afternoon. However, it is also a time when, stuck in the seat which, being at the start of the line, I am usually lucky enough to get, I can look ahead and think about any difficulties that might arise in the day.

Now, on my last Wednesday at the health centre before a week's break, I am thinking about what I will need to do to make my caseload 'safe' and to put the waiting list, for which I now have responsibility, in order before I go away. Emerging from the underground station, I walk towards the familiar and rather friendly sight of the big Marylebone Parish Church. There is the usual heavy traffic streaming along either side of the Marylebone Road: buses, taxis, delivery lorries, cars, couriers on motorbikes and the occasional ambulance or cyclist but fewer people (no tourists yet) than there will be later walking along the pavements. The air is hazy and there is a light mist of rain. I enjoy the fact that it is light and that spring is nearly here. The brief walk is enjoyed for the opportunity to be outside before descending into the crypt for the morning.

### 8 a.m.

I arrive in good time after an unusually straightforward journey of one hour and let myself into the practice as the door is not unlocked until 9.00 a.m. From behind the stacks of files in reception I hear Con's voice and I call out a greeting before settling in to my getting-in ritual, which is a matter of routine by now, allowing my mind to work ahead, beginning to mull over the three patients: Zoe, twenty one, who is on the second of ten weekly counselling sessions, Claudine, a new African patient I'm seeing for the first time and who sounds very troubled, and Ruth, in her eighties, whom I see every five to six weeks in Service D, our intermittent service. These three, and individual supervision with Marilyn, will form my morning.

First, I collect the keys to our tiny counsellors' office which also acts as a storeroom for the practice nurses' equipment and for a heap of old IT equipment that no-one seems to use now. Then I go to my appointments book and the staff pigeonholes to see if I have any messages or letters. I switch the kettle on and go into the dark counsellors' office to leave my coat and briefcase before returning to make a cup of tea.

I am joined at the kettle by Joyce, a locum GP who referred the first patient I will see this morning, Zoe. Joyce thanks me for leaving the notes out for her the previous week, and I confirm that I think Zoe is well motivated to work in counselling and that I will keep her informed about her progress. With my tea, I then continue on my well-worn path back the way I came, stopping by the Counselling Referrals box in reception to see whether anyone new has come in. It is still pleasing to see the pile of white GP Referral Forms without the blue 'partner' form that comes from the patient: the Patient Counselling Self-Request Form. As a result of introducing this second patient's form a few years ago we have been able to reduce the number of DNAs (do not attends) for the first counselling session from over 25% to nearly zero, a procedural triumph at the time. One new referral has come in, matched with a patient's blue application form left the same day; no delay is a good sign. I make a note on the waiting list which is down to three patients. This is good news, and means the new referral I have in my hand, who was unable to tell the GP what was keeping her awake at night, shouldn't have to wait more than a few weeks for an appointment. It is a timely referral. Soon we will be into the pre-holiday period and experience tells us that the referrals will build up quite quickly.

Finally, I pick up at reception my appointments book and the three patient files for the day and after a brief conversation with Con, the receptionist, I set off for my room. This is close enough, just at the other end of the crypt, but the physical distance also represents a psychological journey away from the health centre. As I cross over the waiting area, I put down my mental folder of things to do and people I need to catch and speak to, and allow my mind instead to become attentive, to clear a space for what my patients will tell me.

*8.20 a.m.*

I arrive in the consulting room and take the ten minutes I have left to read through the notes I made the previous week on my first two patients. It's a relief to have a window to my room this year which means I can see daylight and feels like a step up in the world. I take a moment or two to digest the information on the records before walking down the corridor to collect Zoe.

*8.30 a.m.*

Zoe is a white 21-year-old girl who did well at school but didn't go on to university. Instead, she wants to play in a band. She has taken various jobs since leaving school and is now working in a bookshop. She was referred because her temper gets her into trouble and she wants counselling to help 'sort my head out'. She spoke last week about her relationship with her mother, an alcoholic, who left home when Zoe was thirteen years old. She has not been in touch with her since, though her younger brother decided to move out of his father's house and rejoin his mother three years ago. Zoe has a good relationship with her father, but now he has remarried and she no longer has the direct access to him she enjoyed through her teens.

The story is a sad one, of a young woman who is used on one level to having her own way and getting lots of attention to make up for what she has missed. On another level, however, although she speaks of her mother disparagingly and unforgivingly – 'She chose her illness over me' – she knows she misses her and wishes she could have what her friends have: a mother who is concerned about them and checks to see how they are. She is used instead to being older than her years, to putting on her mother's shoes and, in a sense, being the lead singer in the band. However, there is a good deal of spark and intelligence and also, as the GP and I agreed earlier, an openness to thinking about herself which I hope to help her harness.

This is Zoe's second session out of the ten agreed. She tells me it is her birthday this weekend. She is going to see her father and stepmother. Her stepmother is 'all right', she tells me, but she is always the one who answers the phone and Zoe can't stand the way she says, 'Thanks for ringing.' Zoe thinks to herself, 'I'm not ringing *you*,' but she doesn't say it. Instead she finds herself getting angry at work about the 'petty things'.

I note silently that Zoe can't stand having someone coming between herself and her father, and has brought the problem she has with wanting to be Daddy's only girl now that her mother is out of the way. Aloud, I take up the anger she also feels at coming to see a counsellor who is there to listen to her when she has for some time been the adult, the strong one who listens to others. I also say she seems to want to be special to her father, to have a hotline to him almost like a wife. She goes on to describe the choice ahead of her this weekend: she's torn between being a good girl who behaves or being 'a brat'. I say perhaps it's like that here, too. It's difficult and rather hateful to be in the good girl role of 'daughter', or 'counselling client' when she's had to be like an adult for so long. However, if she simply plays a role of either good girl or brat then nothing important really gets spoken about and we can't listen to each other and think.

She looks surprised, then seems to take stock before telling me she doesn't know what to expect from counselling. I try to take the opportunity to establish the shape of what we can and cannot do in our sessions together. At the same time, I feel caught in the cleft stick of being away the following week and needing to address that. She compares counselling to driving lessons and I say she would like counselling to sort things out for her very quickly but float a thought that it might take quite a long time for her to come to terms with things. I don't feel confident that this really makes sense to her but she talks about being lonely and worrying that she will turn into her mother, antagonizing everyone. She doesn't drink because she fears losing control and bingeing. Sometimes she doesn't eat either. She thinks she is really very stuck and is frightened about moving on and 'driving' her life herself. She is used to so much responsibility, and a kind of family status and importance, but somehow she is frightened of many of the things her friends take for granted.

At the end of the session we talk about the fact that I will not be here the following week and she tells me she knows her holiday dates. I note them down and confirm the sessions we have left. Before she goes, she says, 'See you in three weeks then,' and I say, 'No, two,' commenting that it seems a long gap between sessions, when we have just started to talk about things. She starts to say no, she doesn't mind, it will give her a chance to think, but then stops herself and says, 'Yeah, it'll be a bit odd.... In two weeks then, we meet in two weeks.'

### 9.20 a.m.

I take a couple of minutes to let the session settle inside me. I feel a bit worried. Am I trying to do too much in too short a space of time or making it too complex? Three time schemes might be too many for her to hold in mind: the ten sessions we have; the thought of longer term work one day; and the two weeks until we meet again. I wonder if she will come back. Then I remember that she did address the break and give me a chance to get the timing right. That was an important interchange that took place at the door, when so often significant things slip out.

I make a brief note on the file. 'Focus on family situation and particularly rivalry with stepmother, and perhaps with all "mothers". Some worries about herself, particularly about becoming like her mother. Short-tempered at work; avoiding situations where alcohol involved; not eating properly. But using time fruitfully to get hold of her pattern. Will discuss longer term work and ref. for psychotherapy. Next appt. 2 weeks time'.

### 9.30 a.m.

I go to find my next patient, who is not there. I look into reception to see if there are any messages and find a note from my third patient who comes once every six weeks and is due later this morning. She wanted to confirm the time and Jo, one of the receptionists, was able to do this for her. I look in the waiting area of the health centre, in case my next patient is there. The benches are full and I scan the faces, feeling a little like one of the GPs, but she's not there.

I take the opportunity to go into the counsellors' office and do a quick update on the waiting list, which I will have to photocopy later as I will not be here for the bi-monthly meeting of GPs and counsellors next week. I can do this fairly mechanically now so my mind begins to assemble what I know about the new patient I'm due to see next. I put the list ready for photocopying later and go out to the waiting area again. Jo catches my eye and tells me my patient is here, struggling to pronounce the long African surname. I go to collect her.

It is Claudine's first appointment and I am aware from her notes that she has broken several appointments with other members of the team. It says on the file that she has been the victim of a terrible assault by a man some years ago when she was pushed out of a window and both her legs were broken. There are photographs on the file of a black woman whose face is distorted by abrasions and bruises. I have spoken with the referring GP, Gordon, who says she wants and needs to talk about it now. This all makes sense, but I am conscious of some lack of connection within myself which I am not sure about. Is it to do with the many appointments she has missed? Or does it have to do with my sense of anxiety as a white person about an anticipated alienation from her which I need to overcome, about her difference, her colour, her foreignness, each brought more sharply into focus by her French accent on the phone and my horror about the violence that has been done to her? It could be any or all of these.

Claudine herself turns out to be a smallish, attractive young woman. She is distressed at being late and shows me her travel card which had expired, as though she thinks I need to be convinced. I think of the photos in the file and have two thoughts at the same time: that she has recovered well physically and looks very ordinary; and that she's showing me something, as though it's important to her to have a record of things that might not be believed. I find myself wondering if she's showing me what it's like to live in a society where black people generally are often mistrusted and suspected of giving false information.

The story she goes on to tell me is terrible. She tells it in a voice that is shaking. Her eyes keep filling with tears that spill down her face but she carries on, brushing them away with her hand. Her English is sometimes clear, sometimes obscured, by her accent and her emotions.

Claudine arrived in Britain five years ago from North Africa. When she got here the family who were to help her settle into her new country took advantage of her lack of English to carry out a benefits fraud and, when she insisted on going to the Home Office to apply for political asylum, they locked her up in the flat. They made her work as a domestic help and she looked after their little girl for them. She never went out alone. One day they found her trying to make a phone call to the Home Office. Later that day the little girl told Claudine that her stepfather wanted to kill her. That night he came to her room and threatened her with a knife. He then threw her out of their first floor window.

Claudine says she should have died. That was the plan. Instead, both her legs were broken. It was a summer night and some passers-by called an ambulance. The man followed her to the hospital and attacked her again as she slept but was caught and arrested. She stood as a witness against him and he was sent to prison for seven years but was released early. He does not know where she lives now but she's terrified she'll come across him in the street and he'll attack her again. She feels he still wants to kill her.

I have half an hour to digest something of this and to let her know that I'm taking in what she's telling me. I find myself sitting forward in my chair as though trying to imprint my presence on her and, as she is speaking, say with my body, 'I'm listening'. I choose my words carefully.

I say that what has happened to her is dreadful and I need to understand more but I also want to talk about her coming back because we don't have long in one session. I curse myself for booking her in the week before my holiday and say I saw she had signed up on the counselling form for the option of one or two exploratory sessions only but that I would hope she would come back for another session in two weeks time. She nods but I don't feel she's taken it in. I leave it for the moment and ask about her life in Africa.

She tells me her family was dispersed following her father's imprisonment for membership of the government's opposition party. He was in prison for eleven years and was tortured, left blind in one eye and 'ill'. Claudine was ten or eleven years old when he was arrested and her mother had to leave the country for her own safety, so the children looked after each other. Her oldest brother was twenty then. When her father came out of prison he testified to his ill-treatment in prison before an international conference. As a result, the whole family had to leave the country for places where they had friends or contacts. The 'family' she came to here were friends of her aunt and had offered to take her in. She had sisters in Africa, France and Canada and brothers in Russia. Her father was now in Canada and her mother still in Africa but in another country.

The clock is coming up to half past. I say that she must have expected something better when she came to this country but that it has gone horribly wrong. I ask about where she lives now and she says she's in a hostel, that she has friends there and feels secure inside. It's only outside that she feels the fear again. She begins to tell me again the story of what happened when she came here. I say she has told me this and that I remember. She looks at me and goes on to the next part of the terrible story. I say again that she told me this too and that I have taken it in, I remember, but that perhaps she can hardly believe it, hardly take it in herself. I say she went to court and spoke against the man who tried to kill her. I say we do have to stop very soon now but that perhaps it would help to come back and talk some more. She says she's pleased to have talked to me and as she says this, she looks different. Her eyes are bloodshot but she looks more like when I first met her, more ordinary, more composed. She tells me she's studying English and hairdressing and I find myself remembering the message on her answering machine with its French song in the background. I say I don't speak French well and perhaps it's difficult for her to have to tell me about all these things in English, which is not her first language. She says again she is pleased to have talked and that she would like to come back. She takes out a diary from her bag and makes a note in it with a pretty pen with a gold coloured design on it. I say I'll see her then and she says for a third time, on her way out, I am happy to have talked to you.

I feel now a connection has been made. I also feel distressed by her story and quite tearful myself. I am going to be late for my supervision. I shall have to write up my notes later.

### 10.35 a.m.

Marilyn has made two cups of coffee and is waiting for me. I tell her about the session I have just had in an informal way which helps to digest the horror. We find ourselves, like Claudine, repeating the story as if to try and take it in more fully, and talk briefly about how it's almost impossible to take something so shocking in in one go. We also have a lot to do to prepare for the GPs' meeting the following week, which I will not be able to go to. I give Marilyn the updated waiting list to circulate and we run through my caseload so that she can answer a few brief questions. We agree that the patient I have just seen should be given the chance to come for as many sessions as she wants, probably in our fortnightly service over twenty weeks to lengthen the time of support. Even after that she could be seen intermittently over a longer period if she wants to.

The remaining time is spent discussing a referral I want to make for psychotherapy on the NHS. Marilyn underlines the importance of providing a succinct account of the patient's background and difficulties and of the work we have done together. She is more doubtful about the referral but helps me draft a letter that gives an account of this patient's medical history, with its incidents of cosmetic surgery and abortion. I draw attention to the two separate occasions the patient has come for counselling at the practice, and how this time she feels she will be ready to talk 'in the future', and wishes she had been able to talk 'in the past', but still finds reasons not to be able to do so in the present. These are the reasons for Marilyn's doubts, but I believe, perhaps naively, there is a slender thread of motivation, although from my experience it will need to be grasped firmly for the referral to take.

We finish supervision a couple of minutes before my next patient, and I pass her in the waiting area on my way back to my room. I greet her and say I will be with her in a couple of minutes. I put my things back in my room and quickly go to the loo, mentally clearing some space in my mind before going to collect her.

### 11.30 a.m.

Ruth is in her eighties. She looks younger, but I have come to realize that the impression she gives of strength and vigour is born out of frustration and the terribly stressful life she leads. I see her in our intermittent, six weekly counselling slot. Sometimes she can relax and show me how old and tired she feels. She lives with her husband, who has Alzheimer's disease, and her daughter, whom she describes as 'mentally handicapped'. Their care needs are fairly well met and she is a member of a church group that meets once a month to offer each other friendship and support. Otherwise she rarely goes out on her own.

The counselling sessions cannot help Ruth with her difficulties in finding a more regular carer for her daughter, but she can talk about her loneliness and try to sort out the possibilities that confront her. She can acknowledge her fear about having no-one to depend on, as well as her anger that no-one is as dependable as she is. She tells me that when she goes out on her own she feels unsteady, without an arm held out to keep her daughter by her side.

Today, she speaks of her childhood. She thinks she learnt to be responsible at an early age. Her father was a union activist and her mother was loved by the entire neighbourhood for her good deeds. Ruth's husband had been a prisoner of war so she had brought up their two children with the help of his mother, who was very strict. Her husband had returned mentally scarred by his experiences and they had run a shop together. He had depended upon her very much and living where they worked meant she could be with her handicapped daughter. Their son had died fifteen years ago of a heart attack. Her daughter-in-law was still in touch and they had some family in the north of England but it was a terrible business organizing visits. Mostly, she just 'gets on with things'.

It seems to me there is a glow about Ruth today, and I realise why when she talks about a widower in the church group who seems to be taking an interest in her. However, this seems to heighten her quandary about staying in London or moving out. A relative has offered to help her find a place in the North, where she grew up, and where she will have some family nearby, but she fears that something will happen and she'll find herself alone and stranded in a place she no longer knows. I say I think it's difficult for her to accept the opportunities that do occur because she's not used to people organizing things for her. It's difficult not to be the one in charge. I wonder if it would also make her feel her age. She gives me a long look in which the full force of her character makes itself felt.

At the end, she says she sometimes thinks of cutting out the middle man and finding her own more regular carers. I acknowledge that that also means me and that the sessions here are much more far apart than she might want, and also that I'm a part-timer, so that I wasn't there when she phoned yesterday to check the time. This meant she had to accept the substitute care of the receptionist, which though good enough, may also be frustrating. She says she supposes I know what she needs, in a tone that makes it clear that she is somewhat critical of the small offering, so I reiterate that the sessions are far apart. She says they are helpful though, because I notice things about her that her family do not. We make another appointment, this time for five weeks ahead.

Too late, as she goes, I wish I had acknowledged that she would miss me too if she left London. I think, not for the first time, that the intermittent pattern of a session every five or six weeks doesn't lessen the strength of feeling in relation to the counsellor. It's what happens in the sessions that's different. It makes me think of Ritornello form in music. The intermittent pattern of work is so unlike the Sonata Form structure of brief counselling, with a beginning, a development section and a recapitulation/end. The intermittent sessions seem to recur and repeat themselves in some way although slightly differently each time. I made the mistake at first of thinking that counselling should always move things forward, but it's not like that. It's the bits in between the sessions which carry the music of these patients' lives forward. The work of the sessions, as I see it, is to reflect, and sometimes to reiterate. The key thing is that it is not done alone. The recurring sessions also seem to mimic the pattern of a parent's role when a toddler is learning to move away from the ambit of mother or father but keeps turning his head to reassure himself they are still there. Ruth is not a toddler, of course, but she is unsure whether it's safe to move away from what is familiar and the sessions provide her with a minimal space to consider her options, her fears and the obstacles she puts in the way.

*12 p.m.*

I write up this last set of notes and return to the counsellors' office, where I type up the referral letter discussed in supervision, work out when I will next have an assessment session available and make out an appointment letter for the next patient on the waiting list. I then realize that I didn't write up the notes for Claudine. I do so quickly, then sit for a minute or two looking around our office, still feeling the shock of her story and going through what I have done in the morning before leaving.

On my way out I put the three sets of patients' notes that I have seen in the pigeonholes of their GPs and remind reception that I will not be here the following week. Con has gone and Jo the afternoon receptionist is talking to Lucy, one of the massage therapists. I smile at Lucy, remembering a rare opportunity we had to talk to each other on one of the practice away days, then remind Jo I will not be here next week and leave. My presence in the practice is itself intermittent and I can understand how Ruth feels. The discontinuities make it hard work but that is the lot of the part-time counsellor in general practice.

### 12.55 p.m.

I leave the practice via the cafeteria, glad of its proximity. Although tempted by the mint and pea soup, I ask for a sandwich which I will be able to put in my briefcase and eat before my first client of the afternoon at my other place of work. I climb the stone stairs of the crypt and head for the tube. As I stand at the traffic lights waiting to cross the busy road, I look towards Regent's Park and realize that it is a beautiful day. The sky is blue and the sun is shining.

## ON REFLECTION: CONCENTRATION AND CONTAINMENT

*Marilyn Pietroni*

The work of a general practice counsellor is concentrated, in both senses of the word. Resources are limited so counsellors have to concentrate their thoughts and actions into small parcels of time during which a number of roles and tasks have to be undertaken. The counsellor at Marylebone Health Centre is often practitioner, manager, teamworker and supervisor or supervisee all in the space of one three and a half hour session. However, because a clear internal framework has now been established, it mostly becomes possible to concentrate in the other sense of the word: to listen, to reflect and to think.

The development of the counselling framework and the way it has helped to provide a containing structure for some of our complex problems and pressures will be described in the following chapters. The structure enables us to carry out each of our necessary functions without becoming too confused and is a good example of how organizational frameworks held in the mind can sometimes contain anxiety sufficiently for complex work to be undertaken thoughtfully and efficiently.

The stories of our two days show how human blunders and regrets are however an inevitable part of the work of a counsellor, whatever their training and experience. Such regrets are often only recognizable with hindsight. They have to be realized, accepted, hopefully learned from and then 'put away' so that the next patient can be seen or the next task undertaken. In this respect, we have learned much about Winnicott's concept of 'good enough' by observing the GPs' pragmatism (Winnicott 1971).

In their surgeries, GPs have to move on every five to ten minutes to see their next patient who may bring just as much of a contrast to the previous patient as those described in these stories. The same applies with GP home visits. One patient may have called the GP out for an ailment that was not recognizable as minor from the message left but turns out to be, the next may be living alone in the inner city and trying to cope with a terminal illness. The GPs' pragmatism builds upon their earlier experience as hospital doctors who had to prioritize a range of different and demanding clinical needs as part of their basic professional know-how.

Lacking a training in the management of competing needs and demands, as counsellors we had to learn to prioritize patient's needs differently, given our context of scarce resources. The demand for counselling at Marylebone Health Centre exceeds the supply of resources by a ratio of almost 2:1 at present. We have learned over time how to use the half-hour sessions (later to become Service E) with which Marilyn begins to experiment here, and the intermittent service which offers one session every four to six weeks (later to become Service D) as well as how to prepare patients for referral on to psychotherapy. We explain these specific services more fully in the following chapters.

We try to provide a counselling service that respects the needs not only of individual patients but also of the health centre as a resource system. Obviously we do not want to provide everyone with so little that no-one is satisfied. On the other hand, we try to think rigorously about what will be just enough for an explicit purpose.

# Marylebone Health Centre: containing the complexity of inner city life

*Marilyn Pietroni*

At the heart of the Marylebone Health Centre lies a firm belief in empowering people using its services and encouraging them to become responsible for and to take control of their own health whenever possible.

Patrick Pietroni, *Innovation in community care and primary health: the Marylebone experiment*

## SYNOPSIS

The aim of this chapter is to show the Marylebone Health Centre functioning as a whole within its community. A series of clinical examples shows what life is like for some patients in the inner city, and how the multi-professional team at the health centre and the surrounding inter-agency network respond.

The GPs who set up the practice responded to the varied needs of the community with the development of a bio-psycho-social and inter-professional approach: the Marylebone Model. An intricate meeting structure was developed to foster collaboration between different parts of the multi-professional team and inter-agency network.

## THE INNER CITY COMMUNITY

Marylebone is a very mixed community; poverty and wealth exist side-by-side in separate compartments. On one side of the Marylebone Health Centre patch is the affluence of Harley Street, on the other the restricted life of a Baker Street bed-sit, and in the back streets, the anxious deprivations of a bed and breakfast hotel for homeless people, including many refugees. The environment is also one of contrasts: the noise and fumes of Marylebone Road and Baker Street (two of the main through routes of central London), the calm walks and waterways in Regent's Park, the cobbled mews of old stable yards (converted into small businesses and expensive homes), high-rise concrete flats covered in graffiti opposite anonymous red brick mansion blocks, all divided up by the twisting 'rat runs' of rush hour traffic and one way systems that seem designed to baffle the outsider.

The local population numbers 313 208 in the Kensington, Chelsea and Westminster (KCW) Health Commissioning Agency area of which Marylebone is a part. There is an unusually high proportion of elderly people (20% over 65, 3% over 85) of whom many live alone in Baker Street flats that lack basic amenities; a significant number are holocaust survivors. The ethnic community runs at 21% with the main groups being Black African, Indian, Bangladeshi, Asian and Chinese, each bringing their particular health vulnerabilities and expectations. Unemployment runs at about 13% male and 7% female, but strikingly at about 60% in health centre patients who are referred for counselling.

The Marylebone Health Centre has an open door policy towards patient registration which means that the list of more than 6000 patients is not typical for the locality as a whole (Chase & Davies 1991). The practice has an annual turnover rate of 50%; in every thousand patients 250 leave each year and 250 join due to the number of transient groups on the list: business people, students, refugees, broken or disrupted families and homeless single people.

There are many colleges and universities. Students come from the University of Westminster, the Prince of Wales' Institute of Architecture, and the American College in London. Some students from the Royal Academy of Music, across the Marylebone Road, use the Marylebone Health Centre in the crypt for their health care and the church above as their practice and performance venue. Most of these students are new to London (and some to the UK); they have had to separate from all that is home, find their identity and establish a social circle and then fulfil academic requirements. For some this is too difficult and they need counselling help with the transition.

Temporary accommodation is provided by a large number of hostels, short-lease property and bed and breakfast hotels. Nearly 10% of all new registrations at the health centre are registered homeless and 25% are from ethnic minorities, particularly refugees. When the Jarman Underprivileged Area (UPA) Score was calculated on all new registrations in a one-year period, it became clear that the open door policy had skewed the list to those in greater need (Chase & Davies 1991).

## HEALTH AND SOCIAL CARE NETWORKS

Finally, Marylebone Health Centre is part of a network of other health and social services of which it is possible only to mention a few. There are three acute health services with teaching hospitals that provide the full range of in-and outpatient care: St. Mary's, Paddington; University College Middlesex, nearby; and The Royal Free in Hampstead. They also provide the specialized services for elderly people and people with mental health problems or learning difficulties. There are two NHS community health trusts that serve different geographical patches within the Marylebone practice list: Parkside and Riverside; then North West London Mental Health Trust which provides a range of community and acute services. The community health trusts provide community nursing services: district nurses, health visitors, school nurses and allied services such as occupational therapy, physiotherapy and a dietician. Community psychiatrists, community psychiatric nurses and district psychology services are provided from both the generalist and specialist trusts. The network of NHS service contracts, as they are known, that regulate clinical collaboration between MHC and other providers, whether acute or community, are therefore complex. The idea of a service contract, and the ensuing administration and manage-ment of the cost, volume and quality of services, followed the purchaser/provider split introduced by the NHS and Community Care Act in 1990 (DoH 1990).

As a result of recent NHS policy change (DoH 1998a), Marylebone Health Centre is also one of about 27 practices represented in the local Primary Care Group (PCG) serving a population of about 100 000. In April 1999, the PCG took over the commissioning function of acute and community services from the KCW Commissioning Agency and, through its executive, ensures that suitable clinical governance is established. Until that time Marylebone Health Centre was run as a final wave fundholding practice.

The social services department geographical boundaries are not coterminous with the health services. This is a major problem (which needs national attention) and adds considerable complexity to attempts to provide collaborative health and social care locally. Westminster Social Services Department is charged with providing for all client groups in the area. It sets its own criteria for services to elders, people with disabilities, those with HIV/Aids, with learning difficulties, and with mental health problems and children with special needs or in need of protection. It also places annual contracts with its own selected range of flexicare and homecare services, who provide vital domestic help, bathing, laundry, shopping and so on. The social services teams are reorganized frequently, just as the NHS has been, which makes keeping up with procedures, personnel and selection criteria difficult, to say the least. However, the social workers work closely with the practice team, including, in some complex situations, the practice counsellors, as described in Part 3.

Notable voluntary sector organizations are Westminster Association for Mental Health, the Westminster Bereavement Service, Westminster Carers and those services provided (until recently) by the church of St Marylebone itself: Crisis Listening, Befriending, and a counselling service open to all the community and not solely to patients at Marylebone Health Centre as is the one described in this book. The Church Army also has a large nearby hostel for homeless women, and Age Concern provides a good range of day care and other support services.

## MARYLEBONE HEALTH CENTRE: THE HISTORY

The health centre was opened in 1987 in the beautifully converted crypt beneath St Marylebone Church, literally a step away from the pounding Marylebone Road. It has become known for its inter-professional or holistic approach to health and social care. This inter-professional approach is the practice's chosen response to the complex health and social care needs of the busy inner city community.

Collected papers from the first eight years of the health centre's work were published in the first book in this series, *Innovations in community care and primary health: the Marylebone experiment* (Pietroni & Pietroni 1996). The papers describe how orthodox general practice services are offered along-side complementary medicine, counselling, befriending and a community outreach approach.

The integrated approach was initially developed in the late 1970s by Professor Patrick Pietroni, then a family practitioner at the Department of Family Medicine in the University of Cincinnati. There, too, was a large urban community where downtown poverty existed alongside big business and a university. Cincinnati offered an ideal testing ground for a bio-psycho-social approach to inner city stress. Patients who came to the department of family medicine to see the doctor in the usual way with a stress-related complaint or illness, such as chronic pain or fatigue, insomnia or difficulty in concentrating, were referred to the Stress Clinic where Patrick and Marilyn worked together to develop an integrated model from their complementary backgrounds in family medicine, social work and psychotherapy. They developed a six-fold patient education programme which was offered alongside orthodox treatment addressing the following areas:

- the meaning of stress
- the contribution of diet and nutrition
- the importance of exercise
- skills in mental focusing/meditation, breathing and relaxation
- managing life changes, loss and mourning
- understanding different types of psychological defence.

This early six-fold model was further developed in the 1980s at the Lisson Grove Health Centre, London, in collaboration with colleagues at St Mary's Hospital Medical School, notably Julienne McLean, a research worker with a background in medical sociology. When in 1987 the practice moved into the crypt of St Marylebone Church at the invitation of the then rector, the Reverend Christopher Hamel Cooke, a major grant from the Wates Foundation made the full scale Marylebone Experiment possible.

The Marylebone Model of inter-professional care, as it became known, developed rapidly over this period. It reflected the original bio-psycho-social model developed in Cincinnati but now went much further thanks to the appointment of the extended team. In 1987, in addition to orthodox general practitioner and nursing teams, specialist practitioners were appointed in each area of need: a team of complementary health practitioners led by Dr David Peters, a counsellor and community outreach worker Vivien Webber, and a director of research Dr Peter Davies. Thus, the inter-professional model of the Marylebone Experiment emerged and still continues to be developed. It is usually represented as a Flower Diagram with the patient, client or customer (depending on the language framework used) at the centre (Fig. 2.1). The conceptual foundation is based on whole-person care, delivered through sustained inter-professional and inter-agency collaboration, and with an awareness of and relationship to the local and national policy context.

The academic and research environment of the health centre has been generously supported by the charity, Marylebone Centre Trust, and by the University of Westminster, where some staff (including one of the authors) have appointments in the Centre for Community Care and Primary Health. Two of the GPs are also academic staff (Dean and Associate Dean) of the North Thames regional postgraduate system for general practitioner training and continuous professional development, linked with the University of London.

## THE MARYLEBONE MODEL

The art of the Marylebone Model lies in its flexible response to the complex needs of patients in the inner city. GPs have a greater repertoire of responses to patients because there is an extended part-time team available on site about once a week. If a patient comes with a physical problem, it can be investigated and treated in an orthodox medical way, drawing on the contribution of the range of professions at the practice, or by the community or hospital teams described above. If a patient is stressed, physically tense, or suffers from what the complementary therapists call a structural problem, such as back ache or a stiff neck, s/he can be referred by the GP to the on site osteopath. If the patient needs and wants to talk, s/he can be referred to the practice counselling team. If the patient is a refugee, s/he may get some help from community outreach or befriending.

At Marylebone Health Centre, as in any other general practice, the GPs, practice nurses and community nursing team provide the core services on a round-the-clock basis. The different workloads and appointment times are significant because they reflect the pattern of work of each profession as well as defining the opportunities available for liaison or meetings. A GP sees on average thirty patients a day and a hundred and twenty to a hundred and thirty a week for between five and ten minutes each, and provides an on-call service through the local GP cooperative. At the peak of the influenza vaccination period, the practice nurse gives seventy vaccinations a day, with approximately five minutes allocated to each appointment, and an average of three hundred and fifty per week. Each patient enters through reception, including the frequent new registrations. These intensive, daily working patterns of the GPs, receptionists and practice nurses contrast with those of the part-time teams, the counsellors and complementary therapists, and that contrast shapes the rhythm of the week and sets limits on dialogue within the team. It means that Wednesdays at Marylebone Health Centre are practice meeting days because this is usually the clinical day for part-time members of the extended team.

The complementary practitioners and counselling team work mostly a half or one day a week, seeing between four and ten patients a week for up

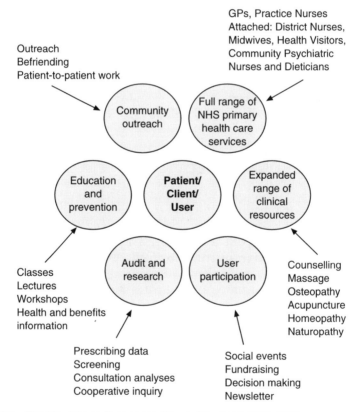

**Figure 2.1**   The Marylebone Experiment. Flower Diagram 1 1987–1992

---

**Figure 2.2**   Marylebone Health Centre multi-professional team

**Clinical team**

| | |
|---|---|
| GPs | 4 FTEs plus 1 trainee and 2 PT clinical assistants or locums |
| Practice nurses | 2 job sharers |
| Osteopaths | 2 PTs (one medical) |
| Homeopaths | 3 PTs (two are also osteopaths and one is also the naturopath) |
| Naturopath | 1 PT |
| Massage therapists | 1 PT plus 1 or 2 students on placement |
| Counsellors | 3 PT recently reduced to 2 PT |
| Community outreach | 1 FT or PT (varies with research grant and worker's orientation) |

**Administrative team**

| | |
|---|---|
| Practice manager | 1 FT |
| Secretary | 1 FT |
| Data enterer | 1 FT |
| Fundholding data | 1 FT |
| Receptionists | 1 FT plus 2 job sharers and 1PT |

| | | |
|---|---|---|
| FTE   Full Time Equivalent | PT   Part-time | FT   Full-time |

---

to an hour each. They provide their specialist services following a referral from a GP, who is gate-opener to the expanded range of clinical resources shown in Figure 2.1. Patients at Marylebone Health Centre are always seen first by the GP and cannot in the first instance refer themselves directly to one of the members of the extended team. This policy reflects the need to coordinate care and manage scarce resources.

Other practices offering an extended range of clinical services sometimes allow patients to make direct appointments with the specialist practitioners, but at Marylebone we do not. There are arguments on both sides. The risk of direct appointments is that priorities are set by individual patients and practitioners, without a coherent policy that attends to key areas of need in the patient community as a whole, such as elders, disabled people, those who live alone, refugees and ethnic minority patients who do not speak English. Coherence of clinical understanding can also be lost as each practitioner works in their own compartment without awareness of the different aspects of need being met by different members of the multi-professional team.

At Marylebone, the pressure on resources is considerable and difficult decisions have to be made centrally about how much of which service can be offered to which patients, drawing on information provided by regular audit. The multi-professional team meets every week and regularly discusses these rationing problems, to which there are no easy solutions, especially when considering how patients need to tell their story and receive a response which has some meaning for them.

## INTER-PROFESSIONAL AND INTER-AGENCY COLLABORATION: TEAM AND NETWORK MEETINGS

The multi-professional team employed by the health centre (represented by the different petals in Figure 2.1) meet weekly in a series of meetings with a monthly and annual rotation. Over time the meetings are reviewed and may be changed but the following description applies to the period of writing. The term team refers to the health centre employed staff and the term network refers to the extended community networks outside the health centre. The term multi-professional is used to describe both the team as a whole and parallel interventions carried out independently by different professions, and inter-professional refers to consciously collaborative work between different professions.

The practice meetings are described in some detail because they give a living picture of the practice at work week by week and show the kinds of issues that have to be addressed. They also show how, in attempting to sustain living links between different parts of the system, the health centre has established some meetings which attend to the needs and development of the whole system and some which attend to specific activities in each part. Each meeting has a different purpose to meet the range of communication needed by the work and to build up the team and the network's mutual understanding.

### Week 1: primary health care team meeting (monthly, one and a quarter hours)

Social workers are invited to this meeting from the two local social services area offices, along with district nurses and attached health visitors from the local community health trust, community psychiatric nurses from the community mental health trust, and (by invitation) representatives of key voluntary agencies. Sometimes the school nurse will attend, and periodically, by invitation, representatives of other key statutory or voluntary agencies such as the Benefits Office or the Church Army.

The purpose of this meeting is to discuss shared cases and the collaboration they require within the health centre, and within and between community agencies. Often these will be patients with special or complex needs who receive a range of community services, as well as having frequent contact with the GP, and sometimes with the practice nurse and other members of the health centre team. The manager of the counselling team attends this meeting regularly, as she tends to carry the more complex cases which come up for discussion from time to time.

The meeting ensures that everyone is up to date, that each is aware of what the others are providing, and clinical aims and outcomes can be discussed. From time to time, a member from one of the local agencies, such as the hospital at home service or the school nurse, will provide a brief talk about how their agency works to foster inter-agency understanding. All cases discussed, and any decisions reached, are noted in a meeting log book for future reference.

Difficult aspects of clinical care can be discussed, as well as any differences of view. The strict eligibility criteria and other policies set by different community agencies can also be explained. For example, the practice is on the border between two area offices in social services, which makes communication very complex when different specialities such as child and family services, mental health, care of elders and HIV / Aids services, each with different working sub-systems, are taken into account. The regular reorganizations change what are already difficult and highly complex systems to hold in mind. The meeting provides a space to clarify and emotionally contain this complexity, especially responses to disruptive organizational and staff changes, and helps protect important collaborative relationships by allowing frustrations and misunderstandings to be examined as they arise.

## Week 2: the process meeting (monthly, forty five minutes)

This meeting is attended by any, and preferably all, health centre clinical staff. The purpose is to explore the emotional impact of the work, particularly any painful or problem areas, and to consider any practice or policy implications that arise. The meeting therefore attends to the needs of both individuals and the health care system and acts as a safety valve. General practice is full of pressures. Patients die, suffer from long term debilitating illnesses or acute pain, are sometimes very demanding and rude, expect or need services that cannot be provided, are often anxious, depressed, angry or confused. Many are lonely. Refugees arrive with horrific histories of torture and loss; elderly people live alone, barely able to manage and with no-one to care; some patients even boast to staff of how they exploit health and welfare services. It is a very mixed bag, and staff frequently face serious moral and professional dilemmas, as well as ordinary clinical uncertainty and impotence, and therefore suffer.

The process meeting is the time and place where they can briefly share and discuss their dilemmas and pain with each other in order to process their feelings. For example, the meeting was invaluable when the patient of a new young GP committed suicide; after an international businessman explained to the practice nurse how he had three homes in different countries but received his health care from Marylebone free by using the address of a friend; and when a massage therapist had to face that there was no more she or anyone else could give to an elderly woman who had survived the holocaust, lived alone after her husband died and telephoned the practice day and night with a range of minor problems. The process meeting allows staff to process their feelings and to recognize that others are experiencing similar pressures. It provides a strong sense of shared struggle and endeavour, with the multi-professional team experienced as a living reality instead of as a set of separate parallel parts. As a result, staff are freed to get on with the work without building up a thick professional skin, or social defence, that would deaden their humanity and make them less able to listen and respond thoughtfully to the next patient that enters their room (Menzies-Lyth 1988).

## Week 3: the academic meeting (monthly, forty five minutes)

The health centre was approved by the University of Westminster as an academic practice base in 1993. Some staff have joint appointments or, like the counselling team manager, are funded by the university. Research projects are also shared between the practice and the Centre for Community Care and Primary Health at the university.

In about eight meetings a year, the multi-professional team explores a common academic theme which is jointly agreed to allow the huge differences in methods and belief within the team to be examined in a disciplined way. One year it was decided that the team would examine the meaning of containment, a word much used and taken for granted until an exchange between different team members revealed significant differences of meaning. The first task was to identify the different meanings-in-use and the second to identify examples of each from the different professions present. A third task was to ground each meaning in a common, everyday language, free of the jargon of professional difference and mystification. The hard work undertaken to reach a common language could then be carried over to other areas of collaboration as each profession gained greater understanding of the nature of their differences. This work is described in Chapter 8.

## Week 4: the staff meeting (monthly, forty five minutes)

So far each meeting described has been attended by clinicians and practitioners only, but the staff meeting is different. Chaired by the practice manager, it is attended by the receptionists, the practice secretary and the data enterers as well as other available members of the multi-professional team. The purpose is to address practical issues about the running of the practice.

Often lack of space is on the agenda. The practice list size has grown exponentially since 1987, and the patient files used are A4 size to allow all practitioners to write in them in sequence, including members of the community services. This allows an integrated and sequential pattern of events to be recorded, showing how each new episode of care begins and finishes, and ultimately giving a lifelong picture. However, such files are almost double the size of the traditional Lloyd George envelope files, and the space around reception is limited. Nothing can change that until the practice acquires more rooms, but sometimes small improvements can be made and noting the frustrations is part of the work. Other typical areas of discussion include the 'bread and butter' of general practice: the efficient management of test results, hospital referrals and new patient registrations.

The counselling manager attends this meeting about once every four months, partly to keep in touch with running issues in the whole practice, and partly to be in a position to ensure that each aspect of the practice's functioning is understood by the counselling team. The idea of understanding the whole in order to understand the parts is not a new one, but at Marylebone it is felt to be very important.

## The practice management meeting (fortnightly, forty five minutes)

This meeting is outside of the weekly Wednesday sequence and is attended by the GPs, practice manager and the manager of each unit of the wider multi-professional team: practice nurses, counselling, complementary practitioners and community outreach. The purpose is, as the name suggests, to manage the practice in every respect: staffing, finance, service contracts, buildings and equipment. It has also had a major policy making function with regard, for example, to decisions about fundholding status and expenditure, and now in relation to changes in the health centre's role and function within the local primary care group (PCG). The practice has joined the local PCG of GPs in Central London which is now responsible for the purchase and commissioning of services for a population of just over 100 000, as specified in the White Paper, *The new NHS: modern – dependable* (DoH 1997).

## Collaborative task meetings (bi-monthly, forty five minutes)

The last raft of meetings takes place in a mid-morning slot on Wednesdays and addresses collaboration between the GPs and each specific part of the multi-professional team. They vary in frequency, depending on need. For example, the counsellors meet with the GPs to discuss their joint work every other month, whereas the district nurses have a special early morning time every week to discuss ongoing care of patients in greatest need, and the complementary therapists have a research meeting every fortnight. Individual liaison still takes place as part of everyday practice, but these task meetings allow policy and practice of joint work over a period of time to be reviewed together.

## Review meetings (three times a year, one and a half to three hours)

Finally, the practice has review meetings where the purpose is to report on the audit from each unit of the multi-professional team, to look at problem areas and to manage changes in policy and organization, now a perpetual feature of general practice. Often these large meetings, attended by all, are rounded off with a social event which adds to the fruitfulness and coherence of the team. When the budget allows, an away day in the country provides the venue for these reviews, usually every other year.

## FLEXIBLE PROVISION TO MEET DIVERSE NEEDS: THE FLOWER DIAGRAM AT WORK

The following examples of collaboration between the GPs and the extended multi-professional team show how the services are typically used by patients. The examples have been grouped according to the different 'petals' in Figure 2.1. To mark the important distinction between full-and part-timers, the examples have been grouped into core team and extended range of practitioners respectively. Each example is GP linked because, as stated earlier, this is how we work at Marylebone, with the GP as gate-opener to a range of flexible resources. Since the counselling service is the main focus of this book, examples of work between GPs and counsellors are given separately, in the following chapters.

## The core team: GP and primary health care team

> **Example 1**   GP and practice nurse
>
> Mr and Mrs Newnham are in their late seventies and are worried about both getting 'flu like last year, because winter is approaching. They make a joint appointment to see the GP and tell him how it is more difficult to look after each other when they become ill now they are growing older. The GP listens to their worries in the ten minutes that he has available, then offers priority vaccinations with the practice nurse. She has a two-tier vaccination list where priority is given to patients like the Newnhams who are most at risk.

The practice nurse job shares a full-time post and is employed by the health centre.

---

**Example 2** GP and district nurse

Letty Babcock's husband died last year after a series of heart attacks. Letty lives alone in a mansion flat, and suffers from cancer of the throat which gives her a hoarse voice. She and her husband were always somewhat reclusive, so she now has few friends and rarely goes out. When she does, her voice tends to put people off. She is frightened of dying alone but finds it difficult to have strangers coming into her home. She was, however, very ill after her last surgery, so the GP asked the district nurse to visit each week to attend to her after care and to spend some time listening to her.

---

The district nurse is employed by the community health trust and not by the GP, but they meet every week at the collaborative task meetings and the district nurse also attends the monthly primary health care team meeting at the practice, where Letty is often discussed because people are concerned about her.

As a member of the community nursing team, the district nurse is attached to several different practices, but works to district nursing protocols developed by her own team in accordance with national guidelines. The professional autonomy of GP and community nurse, and the power-relationship between doctors and nurses more generally, have been the subject of much national debate. However, when collaboration works well, as in this example, such issues fade into insignificance in the joint professional commitment to the patient.

---

**Example 3** GP and health visitor

The O'Reilly family have a complex history. Mr O'Reilly spent three years in jail for sexually abusing his six-year-old stepdaughter and her friend ten years ago. Since then he has moved around the country several times, settling in London again after remarrying four years ago. His new wife knows about his history, but is confident that he has 'put it all behind him now'. Their two-year-old daughter, Mary, is a little overweight but is otherwise doing well.

The GP is aware of the history but is impressed at the way the couple are supporting each other and caring for Mary. All feel that a new start has been made. The GP referred Mary to the health visitor at birth and they now work together to keep a careful eye on Mary's progress whilst making themselves available to the O'Reillys whenever needed. The GP and health visitor believe that preventive work is vital, to support the family sufficiently and lessen the risk of a repeat of what happened 10 years ago. They will watch particularly carefully as Mary reaches the age when her older stepsister was abused, knowing that this will be a time of difficult memories as well as greatest risk.

---

Like the district nurse, the health visitor is employed by the community health trust but meets weekly with the GPs, as well as attending the monthly inter-agency primary health care team meeting. These attached members of the community nursing team share an office at the practice, which also helps communication. Although the team keep their own notes, they also record anything significant in the medical notes, as part of the integrated approach. Health visitor and GP also liaise with social services when there is anything of concern to report.

---

**Example 4**   GP and community psychiatric nurse (CPN)

Laurie is a young woman of twenty nine, a single parent who has been depressed for as long as she can remember. She has been in mental hospital in the past, following several suicide attempts, and is currently on anti-depressants. Her husband left her after the last baby was born. She has three children, Kevin aged two, Marie aged four and Clyde aged six. Her new live-in partner, Kareem, is a refugee who does not speak English very well. They met at the pub about six months ago but do not get on well now, although neither wishes to part. Laurie has put on a lot of weight in the last few months and the children are beginning to look neglected. Kareem is reported by Laurie to punish them severely when they are naughty, by locking them in their rooms and hitting them.

The CPN visits the home regularly to talk with Laurie and her family and is available if things deteriorate. She has put Laurie in touch with a group meeting of other young mothers who have been depressed, but so far Laurie has not plucked up the courage to go.

---

The CPN is employed by the local community mental health trust, and is part of their multi-professional team of psychiatrists, psychologists, psychotherapists, occupational therapists and community psychiatric nurses. She also liaises closely with the mental health team in the local social services department, and attends the health centre's monthly inter-agency primary health care team meeting where Laurie's situation is discussed from time to time. The CPN has a complicated role, which crosses many boundaries and places her as a member of several different teams with different ways of doing things.

## Expanded range of clinical resources: GP and complementary practitioners

---

**Example 5**   GP and massage therapist

Ali Akbar is a businessman who imports and exports clothes and fancy goods. He is proud of his business success and is an important figure in the Muslim community. He is a very private man who works hard and travels a great deal, often leaving his wife and family in England. He has suffered from severe back ache for many years and from time to time the GP prescribes muscle relaxants and pain killers. She has referred Mr Akbar to the osteopath in the past but now refers him to the massage therapist because she will help him to relax more and to learn breathing skills that will help reduce tension.

---

The massage therapist is much in demand and can only see each patient for about four sessions of forty five minutes. She knows that if the massage helps Mr Akbar relax enough to learn some self-care skills, particularly with regard to posture and breathing, he may be able to look after his back and general health more effectively in the future. The problem is that many patients enjoy and respond to the respite given by the massage, but do not continue to use the breathing and relaxation skills afterwards. Sometimes, after a few months, they return with a repeat of the same problems.

---

**Example 6**   GP and osteopath

Mia Pilic is in her mid-thirties. She came to England a few years ago, as a refugee from Eastern Europe, with her husband and two small children. The family are still in temporary accommodation in a bed and breakfast hotel, sharing a kitchen and bathroom with several other families. Overcrowding is made worse by the fact that Mia's mother-in-law also came to England as a refugee, and sleeps on the sofa in the living area. The children have bunk beds in a curtained-off compartment in the parents' bedroom.

Mia is a regular visitor to the GP. She has a passionate temperament so the close living is very difficult for her. Her husband also finds it difficult to show affection and to enjoy a sex life with so little privacy. Mia has a neck injury, sustained many years ago, which gives rise to chronic pain. The GP has been unable to find any drug that will help and prefers for Mia to be seen by the practice osteopath, who also has a training in medical acupuncture. The osteopath has seen Mia on and off for several years. He can sometimes make a difference to her pain, especially when it is most acute. He knows that Mia's main problems are socio-economic, but recognizes that if her neck pain can be periodically alleviated the whole family will benefit. As he says, 'Mia carries the whole family on her shoulders. She is the one who has a job, keeps house and tries to get on with life. Her passion keeps the family going and it would be risky to remove it and to open up her depression.'

---

**Example 7**   GP and naturopath

Shona is twenty one years-old and a business studies student at a local university. She comes from Ghana, is tall and beautiful and dresses with great elegance. Unfortunately she has great difficulty with her diet, and suffers from a number of allergies which give her stomach cramps and rashes. The GP knows that there is not a lot she can do, so she refers Shona to the practice naturopath, who is also a homeopath and osteopath.

---

The naturopath asks Shona to keep a journal of all that she eats and drinks for two weeks, and also to note how her symptoms vary, if at all, during that time. He then suggests some specific dietary supplements to help the delicate balances in her system, and advises her about foods to avoid and combinations that she should pursue. He will only see Shona about three times in the first instance, to establish her new dietary habits, but she will be able to re-refer herself if she needs to do so in future.

## Extended range of resources: GP and community outreach team

---

**Example 8** GP and community outreach worker

---

Jeannie Fisher left home in the North of England to come to London when she was sixteen years old. She lived on the streets for some years, before being given a place in a local hostel where she has stayed for longer than usual. She has taken drugs for many years and supports her habit in whatever way she can.

Although Jeannie is not on the practice list, the GPs have a policy of reaching out to those who do not easily access health care. The community outreach worker has established a regular link with local hostels. The outreach worker advises Jeannie about where to exchange her needles and how to get herself on the single person's housing association list. The worker also offers to liaise with the social services drug team, but Jeannie says she does not want their help and gets abusive when it is suggested. She is very thin and wears ragged summer clothes, even in mid-winter. The outreach worker obtains some good, warm second-hand clothes for Jeannie. She wears these the next time that she comes to the practice, but then reverts to her summer clothes. When asked, she explains that she gave them in part-exchange for her last fix.

---

The community outreach worker keeps in touch with the hostel and sometimes sees Jeannie on her visits there. Eventually she manages to persuade Jeannie to register with a GP, and to come in to the practice to be seen when she has a health problem. The registration is a considerable achievement as Jeannie has remained suspicious of professionals ever since her period of living on the street.

---

**Example 9** GP and volunteer befriender

---

John is in his late sixties and recently widowed. He looked after his wife, who had multiple sclerosis, for many years. She became his whole life. Now that she has gone, he finds it difficult to know how to begin living again. His only interest is in collecting coins. The GP asks him if he would like some company to go shopping from time to time, and he somewhat doubtfully agrees.

Margaret, a receptionist at the practice, is organizer of the practice volunteers and befrienders. The befrienders are themselves patients at the practice who have offered their help to others. They are first vetted, and then sign a confidentiality statement and receive introductory training before providing services. Margaret knows of another widower who is having trouble adjusting to life alone, and asks him if he might pair up with John for an occasional outing. He, too, is uneasy about the suggestion but goes along with it 'to please Margaret'. To their mutual surprise, the men get along well and agree to go to the pub together for an hour every Friday lunch time after shopping. The friendship goes no further but lessens the isolation in each of their lives.

## IN CONCLUSION ...

In settling on the flexible range of services indicated in Flower Diagram 1, Marylebone Health Centre interprets the needs of this very mixed, inner city community in a particular way. By offering this extended range of responses to these typically diverse inner city needs, the health centre not only offers choice to the patient but also gives support to hard pressed GPs, practice nurses and community health services. They know that their difficult tasks can sometimes be shared with other members of the multi-professional team whom they know well and can talk to easily.

In summary, the Marylebone Experiment comprises:

- a bio-psycho-social approach
  - under one roof
  - within easy reach of the community
- the GP as gate-opener to a range of flexible responses
- the core team of GP, practice nurse and community nursing team
- the extended range of interventions: counselling, complementary therapies and community outreach.

# Developing the counselling service

*Marilyn Pietroni*

A benign establishment, therefore, must not be afraid of becoming 'an authority', but it must be an authority that knows itself and in this sense has a capacity for reflexiveness. We might say that its authority should have an 'as if' quality about it. In other words, it should not lose the original quality of playfulness which was so necessary for its own empowerment.

Paul Hoggett, *Partisans in an uncertain world: the psychoanalysis of engagement*

---

## SYNOPSIS

This chapter explains how counselling resources were developed from the employment of a single counsellor to a team of three, following the introduction of a Counselling Volunteer and Supervision Scheme. The scheme also changed relationships in the multi-professional team as a whole, and led to the introduction of the Counselling Referral Protocol at the health centre, with a motivation test in the form of a Patient Request Form. A structured Menu of Counselling Services was then developed, ranging from one session only to a core service of brief weekly or fortnightly work of ten sessions, and a long term intermittent service for more chronically disturbed patients, or those needing long term support for other reasons.

These changes allowed a wider range of patients to be seen in a flexible but disciplined framework, reduced wastage of resources through 'did not attends' (DNAs) on first appointments, and provided greater transparency of counselling activities for audit, research and service development; a wider range of counselling methods also became available.

---

## ORIGINS OF THE COUNSELLING SERVICE AT MARYLEBONE HEALTH CENTRE: 1987–1991

The counselling service began in 1987 when the health centre opened. At that time the sole counsellor was responsible not only for providing the counselling service, but also for establishing and supervising certain aspects of the community outreach and befriending work as shown in Flower Diagram 1 (Figure 2.1, p. 30).

These first five years are described in a paper by Vivien Webber (Webber, Davies & Pietroni 1996), the first counsellor and psychotherapist. She describes the kinds of patients referred, their presenting problems, the number of sessions given and the use of occasional home visits undertaken by an attached social work student. At least two thirds of the patients seen were women, and the emphasis then was on brief work of one to six or eight sessions; DNAs on first appointments ran at around 28%. About 13 counselling referrals were made in each 1000 GP consultations, in contrast to 1.7 referrals to psychiatric outpatient clinics from the same period. GPs varied considerably in the number of counselling referrals they made during the period of study. The main presenting problems were:

- interpersonal relationship problems (45%)
- stress (23%)
- depression and difficulties around life transitions of different kinds, such as leaving home and becoming a student (20%)
- the break-up of a long term relationship, or loss due to unemployment or bereavement (12%).

At that time, the counsellor was considered to be a member of the overall complementary practitioner team, represented in Flower Diagram 1 (Figure 2.1) as the expanded range of clinical resources. This classification may seem strange to some, but the rationale then was that counselling as an activity in general practice was 'complementary' to medicine. The more usual meaning of complementary medicine, as a health intervention of a non-allopathic kind, such as homeopathy, osteopathy or naturopathy, has since been adopted.

The original configuration, which combined counselling and community outreach in one worker, had some advantages, because it allowed the work in the community to be considered alongside the practice-based counselling, and to stay in close touch with what was confronting the complementary therapists. However, it became clear that the centre's open door policy led to more deprived and marginalized groups being served. As a result, the GPs decided that the itinerant and frequently troubled inner city population needed community outreach, counselling, and complementary therapy to be more accurately targeted, and that each type of intervention needed evaluation and management in its own right. In 1992, the extended practitioner teams were therefore reorganized into the three separate units shown in Flower Diagram 2 (Figure 3.1). The author joined the practice at this time, via the university link, working for the first two years as the sole counsellor/psychotherapist alongside Vivien, who now managed the community outreach and befriending services.

A small charity, Marylebone Centre Trust, had been established to help fund research and development. It was the Trust that established the important link with the University of Westminster. A significant research

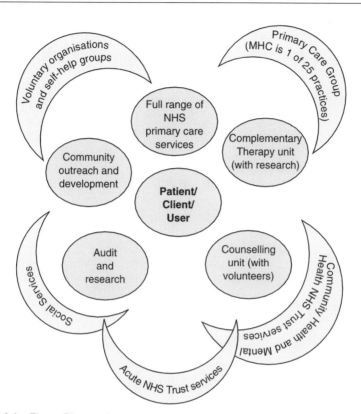

**Figure 3.1**  Flower Diagram 2

profile followed, and an extensive post-graduate inter-professional education programme was launched, building on the work of the centre, just as the implementation of the NHS and Community Care Act 1990 took place. The work of this period is described in *Innovations in community care and primary health: the Marylebone experiment* (Pietroni & Pietroni 1996).

This 1992 reorganization reflected increasing precision in targeting the needs of patients from the local community, based on extensive audit of the first five years of practice undertaken by the research director, Dr Peter Davies, based at the University of Westminster, and one of the GPs, Dr Derek Chase (Chase & Davies 1991).

A conceptual framework for the reorganization was provided by Dr Patrick Pietroni. The matrix of care (Figure 3.2) showed (on the vertical axis) how inner city life was characterized by different levels of distress, which needed different responses (on the horizontal axis) from the health centre's multi-professional team and inter-agency network, including from the patients themselves. Different needs could thus be met by the core primary health care team, by the Community Health Trust, by each of the

| | Communication skills | Information | Befriending | Support groups | Counselling Psychotherapy | Self-care stress management | Community outreach | Massage | Spiritual guidance | Psychotropic drugs | Psychiatric services |
|---|---|---|---|---|---|---|---|---|---|---|---|
| **Human** | | | | | | | | | | | |
| **Unhappiness** | | | | | | | | | | | |
| Loneliness | | | | | | | | | | | |
| Isolation | | | | | | | | | | | |
| Helplessness | | | | | | | | | | | |
| Physical disability | | | | | | | | | | | |
| Chronic illness | | | | | | | | | | | |
| Unemployment | | | | | | | | | | | |
| Homelessness | | | | | | | | | | | |
| Tired all the time | | | | | | | | | | | |
| Frequent attender | | | | | | | | | | | |
| Physical presentation | | | | | | | | | | | |
| Psychosomatic disorder | | | | | | | | | | | |
| | | | | | | | | | | | |
| **Crisis Work** | | | | | | | | | | | |
| Bereavement | | | | | | | | | | | |
| Marital breakdown | | | | | | | | | | | |
| Loss of job | | | | | | | | | | | |
| Loss of function | | | | | | | | | | | |
| Termination | | | | | | | | | | | |
| | | | | | | | | | | | |
| **Psycho-neurotic** | | | | | | | | | | | |
| **Disorder** | | | | | | | | | | | |
| Anxiety | | | | | | | | | | | |
| Depression | | | | | | | | | | | |
| Eating disorders | | | | | | | | | | | |
| Insomnia | | | | | | | | | | | |
| | | | | | | | | | | | |
| **Psychotic** | | | | | | | | | | | |
| **Disorders** | | | | | | | | | | | |
| Schizophrenia | | | | | | | | | | | |
| Manic depression | | | | | | | | | | | |

**Figure 3.2**  The matrix of care

three newly differentiated units, and by specialist agencies, such as the community mental health team.

Patients also organized themselves, with Vivien Webber's help, into a singing group and a befriending network, and a telephone support line was provided by a dedicated patient volunteer for people who were over seventy five and living alone. Patients were further empowered by the appointment of a patient liaison officer, Sybilla d'Uray Ura, funded following the Patient's Charter (DoH 1991b). She worked hard at the two-way communication between patients and professionals which enabled complaints to be heard and the new systems to settle down (Pietroni & d'Uray Ura 1994).

This differentiation of the practitioner units marked the beginning of a move from the 'forming' stage of the early years of the multi-professional team, to the 'norming' and 'storming' stages of inter-professional collaboration, based on a deepening understanding of differences. The way was now clear for the counselling service and each of the other units to develop in their own right.

## THE COUNSELLING VOLUNTEER AND SUPERVISION SCHEME 1993–1996

In 1993 a new counselling system was thus free to develop. A form of counselling apprenticeship was offered to qualified counsellors (or psychotherapists) who were prepared to commit themselves to one year of unpaid work for half a day a week, with guaranteed referrals, in exchange for free on site supervision from an experienced supervisor on the same day. The scheme thus increased counselling resources without incurring extra cost and also provided a career opportunity for counsellors to gain supervised post-qualifying experience. Newly qualified counsellors need to build up a profile of supervised clinical experience for accreditation with the British Association for Counselling (BAC).

Apart from the BAC requirements, why else might counsellors be prepared to work without pay in exchange for supervision? For an experienced and well-qualified supervisor fees are upwards from thirty five pounds per hour on the open market, and suitable vacancies near to a counsellor's home or practice can be difficult to find. It is not unusual for counsellors to spend an hour travelling each way which, with the supervision hour, adds up to virtually half a day a week. It was not surprising, therefore, that the scheme's guarantee of two or three patients to see each week, with free on site supervision, all undertaken in about half a day, was considered attractive by applicants for the volunteer counselling posts, which became the focus of keen competition.

Four one-year volunteer counselling and supervision contracts were offered for two counsellors per year between 1994 and 1996. The scheme increased both the number of counselling hours available to the patients each week, and also the range of approaches. Individual supervision was provided for one hour every two weeks, with joint supervision on the alternate week. The supervisor was also available for half an hour each week for running queries. The BAC minimum requirement is for one and a half hours of supervision a month for every six contact hours, so the scheme comfortably exceeded this low baseline. The supervisor allocated three of her six clinical hours to supervision over each two week period.

Paid counselling or psychotherapy posts in general practice are much sought after, and are usually offered only to someone with substantial clinical experience who, in addition to a qualification in counselling or psychotherapy, often also has a previous qualification in psychiatric nursing or social work. Such staff, therefore, already have valuable experience of the statutory services of the NHS or social services in addition to their counselling or psychotherapy skills. Once they have got to grips with the demands and idiosyncrasies of the general practice setting, it makes sense to use their experience to develop and supervise a team in this way.

## Resource implications of the scheme

*Accommodation*

With the introduction of the new scheme, three rooms were now required on the same day. Rooms are often a major issue for counsellors in general practice, since inevitably they work part-time and the rooms must be multi-purpose. A good discussion of the issue can be found in *Counselling in primary care: a guide to good practice* published by the Leeds MIND Counselling in Primary Care Project (Rain 1997). Rain's conclusions about the minimum requirements for a counselling room are specified in Figure 3.3. Marylebone Health Centre was fortunate to be able to negotiate with its landlord, the church of St Marylebone, to reallocate its existing

---

**Figure 3.3** Accommodation for counselling (after Rain 1997)

Rooms must be:

- prepared before a counselling session (no stethoscope, couch, instruments etc.)
- private and free from interruption (i.e. soundproof and sightproof)
- comfortable (e.g. armchairs)
- light and warm
- signalled when engaged with a sign asking people not to interrupt
- constant: the same room every time with the same patient.

room provision for the extended team, using specially designated rooms offering ideal conditions.

## Counselling approaches

For the patients, the new scheme meant not only that counselling hours increased, but also that a range of counsellors and counselling approaches became available. The Counselling in Primary Care Trust recommends that each practice, and preferably each counsellor, should have more than one counselling approach available to meet the varied needs of the general practice setting. Three of the four volunteer counsellors appointed during the two year period of the scheme were psychodynamically oriented, whereas the fourth had a more cognitive approach.

## Induction and individual development plans

On joining the practice each volunteer counsellor underwent a three week, induction which included sitting in on at least one complete GP surgery, and observing the receptionists at work for one hour. These experiences were written up and discussed in supervision, in terms of what had been learned about the work of inner city general practice, the health centre setting, and the pressures on staff. Then the counsellors were asked to identify the strengths and weaknesses of their own work, and to shape these into an individual development plan in collaboration with the supervisor. This plan acted as a framework for six monthly and end-of-year reviews, and provided material for the supervision reports to the BAC required for accreditation purposes.

## Information systems

Resource boxes were established for the team as follows:

- examples and ready-typed copies of routine counselling letters (e.g. first appointments, cancellations, wait letters)
- a reading box of key articles on counselling and psychotherapy in primary care
- information on local agencies, including counselling and psychotherapy services
- practice and counselling audit and annual reports
- minutes and notes of regular practice meetings.

This resource system was backed up with a shelf of relevant journals, books and policy documents which ensured qualified counsellors were given a measure of autonomy in relation to their own learning, and that time was not lost if a patient cancelled. Counsellors were expected to become familiar with the NHS policy context.

## From volunteer scheme to counselling team

When each one year counselling volunteer appointment was completed, a substantial two-way review was undertaken in supervision. Although there were no funds available from the health centre to make new staff appointments, two of the four volunteers decided that they would like to continue on a volunteer basis for a further year. By that time the practice was able to make a successful application to the health authority for a contribution to one session for each volunteer/counsellor of three and a half hours per week.

In addition, both counsellors provided an extra hour free for administration, writing, audit and meetings. Though far from ideal, this is not uncommon; the literature consistently recommends that about 60–70% of paid counselling time should be spent face to face with patients and the remainder on meetings, liaison, audit and administration. At Marylebone, however, as is now common practice, counselling contracts are only for one year at a time, due to insecure funding from the health authority. This makes longer term clinical work and evaluative research difficult and the high degree of uncertainty generated plunges the practice and counselling team into an annual round of time-counsuming grant applications accompanied by considerable anxiety, which disturbs the work as well as the team.

The counselling volunteer and supervision scheme has, for the time being, been brought to a close. The authors instead decided to commit the experience to print, using a proportion of the supervisor's time to gather material for the book as part of the commitment to the University of Westminster. The scheme, however, provided the health centre with the benefit of two extra counsellors who developed considerable know-how in post. Not only are they now familiar with the health centre and its local agencies, but they also contributed directly to the further development of the counselling service. Alison Vaspe, a psychodynamically oriented counsellor and one of the authors of this book, joined the practice through the scheme, and has recently taken over as manager of the team having been with the practice for over five years. Romayne Jesty, whose work is represented in Chapter 14, uses a more cognitive approach, and has now been with the practice three years. The two other volunteers who joined the scheme left at the end of their contracts to do research and private practice respectively.

## THE COUNSELLING SERVICE TODAY 1996–1999

### Audit: listening to needs and managing resources

The counselling service, like all health centre work, is subject to audit. Each counsellor completes a record of the number of patients she has seen in each quarter, the age, sex, number of times seen, duration, DNAs and so on. This allows a true picture of the nuts and bolts aspect of resource management and counselling practice to be reviewed. It helps link what can seem like a mechanical operation more closely to counselling practice itself if one remembers that the word audit comes from the Latin verb *audire*, to hear or to listen.

Each year, over eighty of the patients referred by the GPs are seen by what is now a counselling team of three, who can provide a total of approximately four hundred and seventy hours each year or a total of ten hours per week (three sessions) excluding holidays. Although, on average, this provides about five to six hours per patient, a more finely tuned Menu of Counselling Services of various patterns and durations was developed, because experience showed that some patients want and need much less, and others need more. We wanted to think more carefully about these patterns, to make them more transparent to GPs and patients, and to create a framework for future research. A six week package of weekly counselling sessions is common in general practice, as noted by Rain (1997) and lamented by Elder (Wiener and Sher 1998). Clinical research has demonstrated, however, that significant work can be done in ten to twelve sessions (Burton 1998, Malan 1976, Sifneos 1972). It was this pattern of an assessment plus ten sessions that we finally chose for our core brief service.

Audit at MHC also showed, and supervision and clinical experience confirmed, that some patients wanted to come fortnightly as they found it difficult to get time off work every week, so a fortnightly service was introduced. Counsellors also felt that not all patients needed the classic fifty minute session, that some could manage well with half an hour, and that these shorter sessions might make it possible for counsellors to see some more disturbed patients on a regular, intermittent basis, rather on the lines of good psychiatric outpatient clinics. Experience of work with the refugee artist, described in Chapter 9, and other similar patients, was pivotal in making this policy shift.

## A menu of counselling services

A Menu of Counselling Services (Fig. 3.4) was therefore introduced, which allows some patients to be seen only once or twice (Service A), some to receive up to ten sessions after assessment in the core brief weekly (Service B) and fortnightly (Service C) services, some to be seen over longer periods of time on an intermittent basis every four to six weeks (Service D), and others to be seen weekly or fortnightly for thirty minutes only (Service E). Long term intermittent work can thus occur within an ordered and managed framework and is less subject to drift. The sixth service on the menu (Service X) is for emergencies. The advantage of offering these, usually

| **Figure 3.4**   The Menu of Counselling Services at Marylebone, 1996 onwards |
| --- |
| (All sessions are 45–50 minutes except where indicated) <br> Service A One or two exploratory/assessment sessions only <br> Service B Brief counselling: weekly sessions of 50 minutes for 10 weeks <br> Service C Brief counselling: fortnightly sessions of 50 minutes over 20 weeks <br> Service D Intermittent: 30- or 50- minute sessions every 4–6 weeks over a longer period <br> Service E Up to 10 weekly or fortnightly sessions of 30 minutes only <br> Service F Don't know <br> (Service X Emergency: not shown on patient request form) |

half-hour, slots is greater flexibility and responsiveness to patients' and GPs' needs. GPs may occasionally make a direct emergency Service X referral for the same week. Such referrals are rare (about four per year) and the service is not abused to by-pass the waiting list. The referrals usually concern patients with a time pressure such as an unwanted pregnancy, as in Example 1 below, or bad news of some kind such as a new diagnosis of malignant illness, as in Example 2. This menu of services was developed between 1994 and 1996, and formalized in late 1996. A further discussion can be found in Lees (1999). Counsellors' half-day diaries had previously provided for three fifty minute sessions per week. A three and a half hour diary could now be stretched to provide for between four and five patients, including the occasional emergency.

Many counsellors may think it is rather an odd idea to offer patients a menu of services at the beginning. How can patients know what they need if they have never been to a counsellor before? Also, it is not unusual for patients to discover that they want more counselling than they had initially thought. There are safeguards here, in that patients can change their contract with the counsellor (within the total menu on offer) by mutual agreement during the first one or two assessment sessions. The advantages are that the published menu of services makes it:

- transparent from the beginning what the counselling team does and does not offer
- clear that resources are limited
- possible for the patient who wants longer term or more intensive help to seek it elsewhere (a list of other services is provided on the back of the counselling leaflet)
- necessary for the patient to think about his/her needs and counselling commitment.

Since the menu has been offered, fewer sessions have been wasted by DNAs and patients come to the first session with fewer misconceptions about what is possible. Patients rarely ask for fortnightly sessions unless intuitively they feel able to work in this way, and then it is often because they recognize that they have problems which are likely to benefit more from the longer contact over twenty weeks. Those rare patients who select the half-hour sessions often do so as an extension of ongoing work with the GP, and are often more seriously troubled.

The menu of services has also provided counsellors with a liberation of a challenging kind. We can now more easily work in different ways with different patients. The routine conventions and assumptions of very brief packages or longer term open-ended once a week work have been stripped away. These new, brief and sometimes intermittent patterns of work reflect the rhythms of general practice itself, which is often the starting point of the patient's expectations of a counselling service in this setting. Long term open-ended work of one to two years of unplanned weekly sessions often provides the base-line model of counselling training and practice, against which planned brief or intermittent work is often seen, quite unreasonably, as the poor relation.

Several monthly commitments further shaped our new system of resource management: individual supervision was eventually reduced and a case discussion meeting introduced; a session is now booked out for audit and to compose a monthly counselling activity list for GPs. Once every two months, GPs and counsellors meet to review specific patients on that list and to monitor how the collaborative systems are working. A detailed view of the annual patterns of resource management made possible by these changes is provided in Chapter 5.

Once the potential for this more planned and precise use of resources was recognized, the existing Counselling Leaflet (Fig. 3.5) was modified, and a Patient Request Form (Fig. 3.6) was introduced to test patients' motivation prior to assessment, and to allow them to indicate which of the services they thought they might need. A Counselling Referral Protocol was also introduced (Fig. 3.7), which summarised the new procedure for GPs and provided information about criteria linked to successful and unsuccessful outcomes. These changes from a more traditional medical model of referral to a partnership model, where the patient plays an active part in initiating and selecting his/her service, are reviewed later in the chapter.

One can ask why a development like this should take over a year to formalize. The reasons lie in the employment structures of counsellors in general practice, which often mean that counselling has to run on a shoe string. At Marylebone, the single counsellor was originally present only two half days a week, of which some time was taken in meetings, and most in face to face work with patients. There was no team of counsellors for debate and analysis, and initially the audit systems were primitive, with data drawn in an old-fashioned way from diary and clinical records at the end of each year. When counselling in general practice is criticized for the lack of an evidence-base for effectiveness, it is important to remember that the work

## COUNSELLING SERVICES FOR PATIENTS

As part of its inter-professional approach to care, the Health Centre provides a counselling service for patients. The fully qualified counsellors work as an integral part of the practice team and maintain confidentiality within the boundaries of the team.

### WHO IS COUNSELLING FOR?

The people who come for counselling are people whose lives have become unsettled and unhappy for many reasons such as loss of a loved one, relationship problems, loneliness, sexual or physical violence or mental health problems, difficulties at work or as a student.

### WHAT CAN COUNSELLING ACHIEVE?

Counselling does not offer solutions to problems or dilemmas or take away painful feelings, but it may help patients to find their own way forward. This is not always an easy process, and those seeking help need to be prepared to make an active commitment to thinking about their problems. The service offered by the Health Centre can only provide brief counselling, so patients who want to work in more depth over a longer period may wish to find a counsellor or therapists from one of the agencies listed on the back cover.

### WHAT DOES THE COUNSELLING SERVICE AT MARYLEBONE HEALTH CENTRE PROVIDE?

The initial assessment session provides an opportunity to consider whether counselling or some other form of help is appropriate; sometimes a referral to another agency may be suggested. Where counselling at the Health Centre is offered, the patient and counsellor discuss together the number of sessions and agree a focus of the work. It is rare for more than ten sessions to be offered due to the pressures on NHS resources. Sometimes only one or two sessions may be required. (See loose page for range of services.)

### WHAT IS THE COST OF COUNSELLING AT THE HEALTH CENTRE?

A contribution of £5 (minimum) per session is requested towards the cost of counselling. Please contribute more if you can afford it. Students, patients receiving benefits and OAPs need not pay although those wishing to contribute are encouraged to do so. Payment is made directly to the counsellor at the end of each session and a receipt is given.

### NON-ATTENDANCE

Non-attendance is taken seriously because it both disrupts the counselling process and wastes valuable NHS resources. If more than one session is cancelled or not attended the counselling time will usually be withdrawn in order to make the time available to another patient. If a session is booked but not attended a contribution is still requested.

### HOLIDAY PERIODS

At certain times of the year (August, April and December), counselling time is less available due to the holiday periods. Waiting times may be a little longer as a result and ongoing counselling may be temporarily disrupted. Patients are advised to see their GP during these periods if waiting is difficult.

### HOW DO I REQUEST AN APPOINTMENT WITH A COUNSELLOR?

If you would like the counsellor to contact you in order to make an appointment, please complete the attached form and post or return it to reception. Counselling takes place on Wednesday mornings and Friday afternoons only. You may expect to hear when your appointment is within the next two weeks after receipt of your form. If there are no vacancies you will receive a letter asking if you want to wait or go elsewhere.

### THE COUNSELLING TEAM

Romayne Jesty - Friday afternoon
Marilyn Miller-Pietroni - Manager, Wednesday afternoon
Alison Vaspe - Wednesday morning

**Figure 3.5** Counselling information leaflet

## COUNSELLING SERVICE

### MARYLEBONE HEALTH CENTRE
17 MARYLEBONE ROAD, LONDON NW1 5LT

## PATIENT'S REQUEST SLIP FOR COUNSELLING

*(Please complete and return in an envelope marked <u>Counselling Service</u> to reception or post to the above address. Please print clearly throughout.)*

DATE: ............. / ............. / .............

MR / MRS / MISS / MS / OTHER: ......................................................................................................

LAST NAME: ..........................................................................................................................................

FIRST NAME(S): ....................................................................................................................................

ADDRESS: .............................................................................................................................................

.................................................................................................................................................................

TEL: (DAYTIME): ...................................................................................................................................

(EVENING): .....................................................................................................................

Appointments are usually made by post. However, please indicate the best time to contact for discussion of appointment by telephone should that be necessary. ...............................................................................

| EMPLOYMENT STATUS *(please tick ✓)*: | Employed ❏ | Unemployed ❏ |
| --- | --- | --- |
| | Student ❏ | OAP ❏ |

GP NAME ................................................................................................................................................

The counselling service is only available at certain times. Please indicate which is possible for you.

Wednesday am (8.30-12.30) ❏      Wednesday pm (2.00-5.00) ❏      Friday pm (1.00-5.00) ❏

Specific times within each half day cannot be guaranteed.

### THE COUNSELLING SERVICES

This section is to help us to plan for your counselling needs whilst protecting scarce resources. Since Marylebone Health Centre can only provide brief counselling, please try to think carefully about your needs and tick below to indicate the service you think you need. If you know you want more than ten sessions you may prefer to make direct contact with another agency to avoid a change of counsellor. On the other hand, if you want some brief counselling the Health Centre Service is the service for you.

All sessions are 45-50 minutes except where indicated.

A. One or two exploratory sessions only ❏

B. One assessment session and weekly work of 4-10 sessions ❏

C. One assessment session and fortnightly work of 4-10 sessions ❏

D. One assessment session followed by one session every 4-6 weeks over a longer period ❏

E. Up to six 30-minute weekly or fortnightly sessions ❏

*Thank you for helping us to plan your counselling. If after an assessment, it is found that you need a different service from the one you have indicated above, it is usually possible to change.*

| FOR OFFICE USE ONLY: | |
| --- | --- |
| DATE FORM RECEIVED........................................ | DATE OF ASSESSMENT ................................................... |
| COUNSELLOR:    AV      RJ      MP | SERVICE AGREED      A      B      C      D      E |
| £5 OR NO CONTRIBUTION: | DATE OF COMMENCEMENT OF SERVICE ............................. <br> (if different from assessment) |

**Figure 3.6** Patient request form

**Figure 3.7** Counselling referral protocol for GPs with guidance on outcome criteria

*GPs*
- GP assesses in one session that patient needs to talk to someone in the counselling service
- GP has in mind criteria for successful outcome and those associated with failure (listed below)
- GP asks the patient back for a second appointment to prepare the ground and explore the following:
  — patient's reaction to the idea
  — patient's motivation
- GP also explains that:
  — there will be a short wait of up to 2 weeks
  — if it is going to be longer, there will be a 'wait letter' sent by the counsellor
  — counselling is only available on Wednesday and Friday afternoon
  — a contribution of £5.00 per session is requested, unless unwaged
  — patient can indicate preference from menu of counselling services at MHC or find service elsewhere from list on reverse of information leaflet (see below)
- GP assesses whether to give the patient the counselling information leaflet and patient request form in first or second session
- Patient completes patient request form and sends or leaves it at reception (who leave it in the green box)*
- Only after second session, GP completes GP referral form and places it in the green counselling referral box in reception*

*These two items provide audit data

*Counselling Team*
- Referrals will be reviewed and allocated weekly on Wednesdays
- Action will only be taken after *both forms* have been received
- Counsellor's response to referral will be communicated to referring GP
- Notes will be placed in referring GP's tray after each counselling appointment
- Overall list of patients in counselling, indicating service, DNAs etc. is circulated to GPs monthly for information

Menu of counselling services (see Fig. 3.4)

*Criteria associated with effective outcome*
- demonstrated motivation
- an understandable and agreed focus for counselling
- a capacity to use and work in words
- psychological-mindedness.

(Drawn from a wide span of literature (Malan 1963, 1976a & b, 1979 with follow-ups over twenty years, Mann 1973, Sifneos 1972, Corney & Jenkins 1993, Elton Wilson 1996 and the extensive reviews conducted by the Counselling in Primary Care Trust)

*Failures in counselling in general practice*
The Counselling in Primary Care Trust (Curtis Jenkins 1992) identifies the following reasons for the failure of counselling in general practice:
- different concepts of care: the bio-medical (GP) and psycho-social (counsellor)
- patient's attitudes: expecting a cure from the counsellor
- patients' fears that a counselling referral means they are 'going mad'
- GPs use counsellors as a dustbin for 'heartsink' patients who do not themselves want counselling
- counsellors move out of their clinical role to become 'nanny' to the practice
- small premises and/or insensitive receptionists expose counselling referrals in the waiting room and break confidentiality
- fear of placing counselling on life/medical assurance assessment forms
- poor, insufficient or inappropriate training of counsellors in general practice.

takes place in fragile and fragmented conditions such as these, where the survival of annual funding is a key issue.

This chapter now goes on to review the two models of delivering the service represented in the different phases of development.

## THE TWO MODELS: A REVIEW

### The traditional referral model: 1987–1994

The referral process for counselling at Marylebone Health Centre between 1987 and 1994 followed a traditional medical model. The GP filled out a referral form devised by the counsellor (Fig. 3.8), after discussing the referral with the patient and obtaining his/her agreement. The counsellor, on receipt of the form, would then phone the patient or write with an appointment within the next week or two. Where a longer wait was necessary, the patient would be sent a 'wait letter' with a reply slip to indicate whether s/he was prepared to wait for up to eight weeks or wished to be taken off the referral waiting list (Fig. 3.9).

This traditional model mirrors the pattern of GP referral to any other specialist service, such as a hospital outpatient appointment. It is, however, top of the Counselling in Primary Care Trust's list of reasons for failure of counselling in general practice (see Fig. 3.7). When this model was in use, the GP took the lead and the patient consented or not to the treatment plan, and could easily remain a passenger in a communication system carried out in technical language between professionals. A system like this, which could easily over-medicalize an all too human problem and which was often born out of pressure of time, tended to undermine the espoused bio-psycho-social model of the multi-professional team at the centre and disempower the patient; it also lessened his/her responsibility for the process of his/her own care from the beginning.

Since much counselling is about enabling the patient to discover new ways of bearing and negotiating personal responsibility, such a system was clearly undersirable. It also failed to test the one selection factor that all counselling and psychotherapy outcome research is agreed upon, namely the patient's motivation. In the traditional medical model the patient is not called upon to play any active part in seeking counselling, except to agree with the GP that a referral can be made. S/he may do this to please the GP, as an expression of how s/he felt at that moment (but not subsequently), or as a way of leaving the GP consultation and avoiding further uncomfortable discussion. For many patients, the suggestion that they should talk with someone other than the GP is experienced as a rejection, or as being 'palmed-off' with a colleague. They may agree partly to conceal their disappointment and attachment to the GP, who can often be a significant figure in their lives. Establishing a referral system is therefore a complex

**November 1997 Revision GP Form**

Audit
Counsellor                          Date of First Appt:-
Type of Service:-                   A  B  C  D  E
Closed:-                            Number of sessions
Referral on to:-

### REFERRAL FOR COUNSELLING: GP FORM

(Please complete the following information when referring a patient for counselling and make
sure that the patient knows there is a £5.00 contribution except for those on Income Support.)

Name: ...................................................           Tel No: .............................................

Age: ...........................................................

Other Family Members (if any): ................................................................................................

..............................................................................................................................................

Date of referral: ..........................................................

Current Medication (please specify doses):

Number of attendances at MHC in last month: ......................................

Other MHC Practitioners currently or previously involved:

Reason for Referral:

Previous counselling or Psychotherapy (state where, when, for how long and with whom):

Psychiatric History (if any known):

Name of Referrer: ......................................................................

GP's Contact Number and best time to call: .......................................................................

**Figure 3.8**  GP referral form: side one

business, in which there are important issues to consider from three different points of view: patient, GP and counsellor.

The traditional referral method was recognized to be unsatisfactory at
Marylebone for some of the reasons outlined above, which were reflected
in the early years in a high rate (25–30%) of DNAs on first appointments.
Closer audit of counselling activities during the Counselling Volunteer and
Supervision Scheme sharpened the rationale for change. The wastage of

COUNSELLING REFERRALS:  CRITERIA FOR <u>BRIEF</u> WORK
(evidence-based: Malan 1976)

1.  MOTIVATION

2.  A FOCUS FOR WORK / AN 'UNDERSTANDABLE' PROBLEM AREA
(ie, not diffuse, or vague and 'mobile' problems)

3.  PSYCHOLOGICAL-MINDEDNESS:  a preparedness to think psychologically
(ie, not somatisers)

4.  CAPACITY TO USE WORDS (rather than body, excessive silence, etc.)

5.  ALL AGES, RACES, SEXUAL ORIENTATIONS etc.

6.  CLINICAL SYNDROMES / PRESENTING PROBLEMS

"Internal":-  Depression with a focus / reactive
Anxiety with a focus / reactive
Phobias
Severe Mental Illness in remission
Parasuicidal behaviour
Self-harm
Self control problems
Alcohol Abuse - selectively

"External":-  Bereavement / Loss
Relationship problems
Sexual problems
Fertility problems
Unemployment / Redundancy / Retirement
Abuse or post-abuse problems
Serious physical illness
Transition problems (eg, students)
Refugee / Displaced Person problems
Financial problems
Housing problems (selectively:  we do not do social work)
Domestic Violence problems
Harassment problems
Carer / Dependant problems
Study problems

**Figure 3.8**   GP referral form (*cont'd*): side two

resources became clearer when first appointments tripled with the introduction of the scheme. Discussion in the expanded counselling team, following the results of two six monthly audits, led to the development of the new referral system which works much more effectively.

## The motivation test and counselling referral protocol: 1996–1999

The one unequivocal research finding in relation to effective counselling or psychotherapy outcome is the importance of the patient's motivation (Malan 1976, Rain 1997). In early 1996, when the new referral process was

MARYLEBONE HEALTH CENTRE
17 Marylebone Road London NW1 5LT.
Telephone 071 935 6328
Fax 071 224 2924

Date as postmark

Dear

Re: Counselling Request

Thank you for your request for counselling. Usually we are able to respond with an appointment within a few weeks but I regret that on this occasion there have been too many requests in a short period of time and we are unable to do so. It will now be at least eight weeks before we can send you an appointment.

If you wish to wait, please fill in the form below and we will respond when a vacancy becomes available.

Alternatively, may I remind you that other counselling facilities are available outside of the Health Centre which you may wish to consider. The telephone numbers are listed on the back of the blue Counselling Information Leaflet that was given to you by your GP.

Yours sincerely,

Marilyn Miller-Pietroni
Counsellor and Psychotherapist

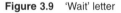

Name
Telephone numbers (day and evening)

I would like my name to remain on the waiting list for brief counselling. I realise that there will be at least 8 weeks wait before an appointment can be sent.

Date

Signed

**Figure 3.9** 'Wait' letter

introduced at Marylebone that increased the patient's role in the referral process through the introduction of a motivation test. The original GP Referral Form (Fig. 3.8) was retained but the new Patient Request Form (Fig. 3.6) was introduced. A new accompanying Counselling Information

Leaflet provided information about the extent and limits of the counselling service at the health centre in various languages (Fig. 3.5). A simple Counselling Referral Protocol (Fig. 3.7) was also developed, which was placed (with a sample copy of the two forms and the information leaflet) with other health centre protocols in every GP consulting room. A protocol is a written system of practice that is agreed and conformed to by all parties, and is subject to regular audit and review. It usually reflects a commitment to evidence-based practice, i.e. practice based on research findings.

The Counselling Referral Protocol provided GPs with guidelines for the use of the two forms and the leaflet, and on the reverse side offered criteria associated with successful counselling outcomes and reasons for failure. Marylebone Health Centre has a series of different GP training and development commitments to fulfil in the region, and from time to time is obliged, on account of staff training and sickness, to use locum GPs. The new protocol therefore provided a simple way of communicating with these part-time staff who were rarely at the practice on the same day as the counsellors.

Research has shown that, in addition to the criteria listed in Figure 3.7, a certain kind of working compatibility between counsellor and patient improves outcome. However, as the Marylebone Health Centre team is small and the available hours limited it is not usually possible to accommodate this criterion unless there is a rare choice of counselling vacancies.

The Counselling Referral Protocol requires that the GP normally sees the patient at least twice before making a referral for counselling. On the first occasion s/he notices that the patient needs to talk more than the usual ten minute GP session will allow, and asks the patient to make a further appointment. S/he gives him the counselling leaflet and the patient request form to read and think about. If the patient makes that appointment, the GP then enquires what thoughts s/he had about counselling and works out with him/her whether a referral is appropriate. Only then does the GP complete the GP referral form (Fig. 3.8), which is placed in a confidential counselling referral box at reception.

If the patient, once having read the information leaflet, decides to proceed, s/he completes the patient request form, which is blue for quick recognition, and sends or hands this in a sealed envelope to reception. The referral box is cleared every week, but a counselling appointment is only sent after both GP referral and patient request forms are received. A reply to the patient is guaranteed in a maximum of two weeks.

Where there is a spate of referrals, as usually occurs at holiday periods, a 'wait letter' (Fig. 3.9) is sent to the patient, indicating that there may be a wait of up to eight weeks before an appointment can be given. The patient is asked to complete a reply slip indicating whether or not s/he still wants an appointment to be sent. If no reply slip is received, the patient is sent a further 'nudge' letter when s/he is near the top of the waiting list, asking him/her to contact the practice within the week if s/he still wants an appointment. If s/he does not do so, his/her name is removed from the waiting list.

## Reducing DNAs on first appointments

It is a research finding of some note that in the eighteen months after the new protocol with the dual doctor and patient referral system was introduced, almost one third of the GP Referral Forms were not matched by a blue Patient Request Form. Those patients were therefore not sent a counselling appointment. This figure almost exactly matches the original audited rate of DNAs on first appointments, in response to which the motivation test of the patient request form was introduced. At the time of writing, DNAs on first appointments stand at only 1%, which has given rise to considerable celebration. The complementary therapists are considering introducing a similar system. The increased preparation for counselling provided by the two GP appointments, backed up by printed information, also responded to Webber's finding (1996) that DNAs on first appointments followed poor GP preparation.

To facilitate regular review of referral patterns, the counsellors circulate a list of their activity on current patients and their waiting-lists once a month, together with a list of any DNAs. This information acts as a useful quick guide to GPs on the outcome of their referrals, the current waiting list, and the progress of current patients in the system. It means that if, as now happens rarely, a patient does not arrive and yet has not cancelled, the GP has a chance to explore why, and to explain that resources are limited and a cancellation is preferable.

For a counselling referral to take root, and for the patient to make it to the first counselling session and then to use the time effectively, motivation, availability and the capacity to bear psychological pain must go hand-in-hand with good preparation by the GP and appropriate information about the service.

## Implications for the multi-professional team

There is no doubt that the critical mass of the expanded counselling team also established a more powerful sub-group within the multi-professional team of the health centre, and provided a useful forum for thinking things through and for forward planning. The innovations that resulted were welcomed by other members of the team, and ensured that the new counselling sub-group was not experienced as a defensive bloc, but rather as a new source of ideas about inter-professional collaboration and maximizing the use of scarce resources. The counselling team had now consolidated its professional identity in the multi-professional team in a positive way; this would have been much more difficult for an individual working one day a week to achieve. The different personalities, methods of work and previous experience of team members were also enriching to the service, and this is worth considering when choosing between increased hours for one counsellor or appointing additional staff.

Organizations go through different stages of development in much the same way as individuals. In 1995–1996, it was as if the whole Marylebone Health Centre organization had reached a stage in development when differences of practice, language and belief between the professional subgroups could be articulated more accurately. These changes are reflected in the work that became possible in the academic meetings during this period, which are discussed in more detail in Chapter 8.

## The menu of counselling services at work: two examples

Two brief examples of counselling work now follow to complete the overview of services in the health centre's multi-professional team and to show the kind of work undertaken by the counselling team. More detailed examples follow in Part 3.

---

**Example – Catrina**    GP and counsellor (Service X, emergency)

Catrina came to London for work. She was twenty four years-old and pregnant, having waited too long to take the morning-after pill. When her young woman GP wondered what that wait might have been about, Catrina burst into tears and explained that she had had a termination of pregnancy the previous year which she had since regretted. She had been unable to tell her parents, had become depressed and felt unable to maintain any relationship for very long. She did not want to stay with her latest boyfriend, but after they had had unprotected sex she stayed in bed watching television to stop thinking.

The GP suggested that Catrina might like to talk things over with the counsellor some time in the next few days and she hesitantly agreed. She was referred as one of the rare emergencies (Service X) and was given an appointment for two days later. In two thirty minute sessions with the counsellor, over the next two weeks, Catrina thought back over the earlier termination and was able to tell her mother about it. She then decided to have a second termination and, having worked on a little of her guilt and self-hatred, she reconnected with her family and felt less depressed. She felt it was unlikely to happen in the same way again, now that she had put the first pregnancy to rest. She was offered and accepted one further appointment a few weeks after the termination.

---

This carefully measured response to a specific problem met Catrina's needs but took only three sessions over a four week period. The appointments were scheduled in the same weekly hour in the counsellor's diary as two other patients seen on an intermittent basis (Service D) over a longer period. The flexibility of rotating appointments in this way allows one counselling hour to sustain three or more patients, including the occasional assessment or emergency.

---

**Example – Zita**   GP, counsellor and massage therapist (Services B and C)

Zita had ovarian cancer which had been treated with surgery and two periods of major chemotherapy that left her sick and exhausted. Her right leg had swollen with lymph oedema and she had become very constipated since the cancer had spread into the bowel. She was single and lived alone in a bed-sitting room, having been a secretary all her life. She gave the appearance of being very ordered but had a strong spiritual life and had become very interested in alternative medicine. She read a lot of New Age literature and regretted not having come across these ideas earlier in her life. She had chosen Marylebone Health Centre because of the range of alternative and complementary therapies on offer.

She had had psychotherapy in the past on a private basis, but now had become unable to work and was living on a small income. She was referred to the counsellor during one of her remissions, to give her support and a space to reflect on her life and her far flung family in particular. First she was seen for 10 weekly sessions (Service B). Her chosen focus was on her complex family relations, and she insisted on pushing her illness to one side.

She was referred again after her illness recurred and now chose fortnightly sessions over a longer period (Service C). She knew this time that she was dying, but referred to the fact only obliquely. As she was so physically uncomfortable, the counsellor discussed with the GP whether lymphatic drainage massage might help, or whether some soothing massage of her extremities and neck and shoulders was all that was appropriate at this late stage.

As Zita became immobile, the GP arranged for a massage therapist to visit her at home several times to soothe her and help her to relax. The counsellor continued to talk with Zita during appointment times on the telephone, and made one home visit at a particularly difficult time towards the end of her life. Two weeks later Zita died quietly at home, avoiding the further hospital admission that she had dreaded.

---

Occasionally, a complementary therapy practitioner will be involved in providing services alongside a GP and counsellor. Usually this doubling-up is avoided, to ensure the scarce services reach as many people as possible, but occasionally, as in the following example, there is a clear need for a multi-faceted approach. We discuss this issue in more detail in Chapter 4.

This was a measured and thought-through response to a patient's exceptional needs in the inner city where she lived and was to die alone, and where the members of health centre team were her centre of gravity and main social contact.

It is obviously extremely rare for a counsellor to do a home visit, but we have chosen this example to show that, at some point, basic assumptions almost always have to be questioned when counselling in general practice. A recent article (Firth & Rowlands 1997) referred to a pilot study on the attachment of psychiatric social workers (PSWs) to general practice, found to be useful because they were trained to provide a combination of counselling and practical help. Although most patients in Firth's study were seen at the practice, home visits were sparingly used to good effect. Few counsellors are trained PSWs, but their professional role in general practice is a neighbouring one and there are occasional overlaps.

## IN CONCLUSION ...

To some people, general practice may seem a somewhat inhospitable climate for counselling, with its pressure on resources and team accountability through audit. In some ways, this is true. To work in general practice, one needs to be excited by and interested in the idiosyncrasies of the setting and the opportunities and constraints it provides in its own right, and not to feel constantly that it falls short of some more ideal conditions. It is possible to do good brief and long term work, but as the stories in Part 3 will show, it is long term work of a particular kind. The disadvantages of resource constraints are offset by the value of being so close to the patient's first point of contact with the GP. Those who have worked in a specialist agency, or in private practice, will find the types of referrals made by the GP at the point of frontline service delivery quite different in nature. They are more immediate, often the needs are raw (rather than pre-cooked in the process of referral), and sometimes they are unexpectedly challenging.

# 4

# The counselling service at work

*Marilyn Pietroni*

The general practice setting is one of the most challenging environments in which to provide counselling. As the principal providers of primary health care, general practice teams offer first contact, ongoing and comprehensive health care to people irrespective of their age, sex or presenting health problem. A very high proportion of the people presenting in general practice have emotional or psychological difficulties enmeshed within a complex tangle of physical and social problems.

Bonnie Sibbald, Foreword in *Counselling and psychotherapy in primary health care*

## SYNOPSIS

This chapter shows key aspects of the counselling service at work. A brief discussion of the audit context is followed by a number of working examples illustrating some implications of the multi-professional perspective at Marylebone. Assessment and supervision issues are considered, and counselling records and confidentiality, controversial areas in the literature, are illustrated with brief examples. Finally, the professional management and insurance systems as they operate at Marylebone Health Centre are explained.

Our picture is a local one. Rain (1997) and Burton (1998) provide an excellent discussion of the issues seen from a national level.

## REFERRALS: THE AUDIT CONTEXT

Counselling referrals raise questions not only of the patient's motivation, availability and suitability; they are made in a context where clinical assessment, audit and resource management have to go hand in hand. We have to consider the costs to and meaning in the health care system of each episode of work, in addition to the more immediate stated needs of each individual patient and our own professional interests.

All Marylebone Health Centre clinicians routinely keep data on the age, sex, ethnicity, postal codes and attendance patterns of patients, including DNAs (did not attends), cancellations and lateness. These data are reviewed in a practice meeting three times a year, when there is helpful pressure from the multi-professional team to use the findings productively in order to understand and improve the services offered. The counsellors' introduction of a motivation test to eradicate DNAs on first appointments, for example, described in Chapter 3, stimulated other units in the team to consider doing the same; GPs also had to reflect on the quality of their preparation of patients for such referrals.

Problem-oriented and clinical assessment data are also regularly audited. In a recent health authority contract for one of the Marylebone Health Centre counsellors, the following clinical categories were listed for annual audit:

- stress
- anxiety
- depression
- interpersonal problems
- bereavement or life changes.

These broad and practical categories were based on earlier annual returns from the counselling services in the area of Kensington, Chelsea and Westminster Commissioning Agency, and we found them fairly workable at the referral and assessment stage and after counselling was completed. They are expressed in simple language and are the types of categories to which both GPs and counsellors can relate. The categories are, however, changed over time by the health authority and are by no means inclusive of all the types of referrals made or acted upon. They were set up before the CORE (Clinical Outcome in Routine Evaluation) outcome measures were established at the University of Leeds (see Fig. 4.1).

The counselling team developed these broad categories into a more detailed system of internal and external problems. The former link to the clinical diagnosis and refer to the patient's psychological state and behaviour, and the latter relate to the presenting problem, often expressed in social as well as psychological terms (such as unemployed). The two groups of categories reflected the bio-psycho-social model of Marylebone. More detail is given in Chapter 5, which gives the annual picture.

Audit data have been collected on these lines for annual review at the health centre for the last two years, and have been useful for developmental discussions with the GPs, as well as in the counselling team, about which patients are being referred and why, and what is happening to them in and after counselling. However, all audit and clinical categories have their limitations and are interpreted differently both by those who provide the data and by those who analyze it. Burton (1998) provides an informative and thorough discussion of the issues. Further discussion can be found in Keithley and Marsh (1995), Tolley and Rowland (1995), and Wiener and Sher (1998). There is no point in collecting data for the sake of it; there has to be a clear reason and significant time needs to be given to training those who provide the service as well as those who analyze and use the data. Mostly this time is simply not available. The counselling context at health

**Figure 4.1**  Outcome measures and selection criteria associated with effective outcomes (See Burton 1998 for an extended discussion of outcome)

The following selection criteria have demonstrated links with good outcome over a wide range of studies over a long period of time and are currently used at the health centre:

- demonstrated motivation
- psychological-mindedness
- a capacity to use and work in words
- an understandable and agreed focus for counselling.

The CORE standardized outcome measure, to be introduced at the centre in 1999 (CORE System Group 1998), is available in long (34 item) and short (17 item) versions from the Psychological Therapies Research Centre at the University of Leeds, and includes sub-scales on the following:

- subjective well-being (current distress and self-esteem)
- symptoms (depression, anxiety, trauma, physical manifestations)
- life/social functioning (relationships, work/leisure, quality of life)
- risk/harm to self and others.

*The Health of the Nation Outcome Scale* (HoNOS) (Wing, Curtis & Beever 1996) has been drawn upon by the CORE outcome measures and is also influential nationally. It includes 5 point scale measures of the following:

- overactive, aggressive, disruptive behaviour
- non-accidental injury
- problem drinking or drug-taking
- cognitive problems
- physical illness or disability problems
- hallucinations or delusions
- depressed mood
- other mental/behavioural problems
- relationship problems
- daily living problems
- occupation problems.

authority level is often one of short term research and audit contracts, and at the practice level of yearly counselling contracts of a very part-time nature.

At present we do not have the staff to undertake any formal outcome studies on counselling at Marylebone, apart from a trigger for reflection in the form of a three point counsellor's rating scale: improved, no change, worse. We also collect data that will enable us to measure changes in medication before and after counselling, as well as the frequency of contacts with the GP. We have provided GPs with the criteria associated with successful and unsuccessful outcomes outlined in the previous chapter. We keep resource management strict, on a case by case basis, but have not yet evaluated outcomes on a series over time.

It is rare to be able to do outcome studies without extra resourcing. Hopefully, greater rigour will be achieved with our forthcoming introduction of the national counselling audit database, CORE, the Clinical Outcome in Routine Evaluation system developed by the Psychological Therapies Research Centre team at the University of Leeds with the support of the Counselling in Primary Care Trust. The picture will always be complex because audit categories interact with clinical judgements and language use and are influenced by different views about the appropriate use of counselling resources. The following typical referrals illustrate this complexity.

## Typical referrals

Experience has shown that notwithstanding the counselling protocol requirement (Fig. 3.7, Chapter 3) that there should be a 'focus' for work, and audit categories constructed locally and nationally, referrals rarely fall into one convenient diagnostic or problem category. Rather, several problems and potential clinical diagnoses, referred to in the technical literature as co-morbidity, tend to combine in a current focus. It seems likely, but has not been proven, that this complexity is related to the inner city context. The following examples therefore show the complex inter-agency approach of Marylebone Health Centre at work.

The second example illustrates more clearly the dilemma for the GP about whether to make a referral to the complementary therapists or the counsellors. Sometimes it is appropriate for a counsellor to cross-refer to a complementary therapist where the patient requests, the GP agrees or the counsellor assesses that a joint approach would be particularly useful, as in the following example.

Two examples, Sheila and Hassan, illustrate a joint approach, drawing on therapeutic interventions from the counsellors and complementary therapists in addition to the GP, which is unusual, mainly because it inevitably concentrates more services on fewer patients. Used selectively and sparingly it can, however, help to produce the critical shift that enables a patient recover the capacity for self-help. There are some situations, however, where a joint approach between GP, counsellor and complementary therapist is more commonly called for (Fig. 4.2). Some examples of this collaborative work now follow.

---

**Figure 4.2**   Doubling up: conditions for collaborative work between complementary therapists and counsellors

- Terminal care
- Bereavement
- Chronic pain and loneliness
- At a point of transition from physical pain to mental pain.

**Example – Lisa**    Multiple problems

Lisa is in her mid-twenties and has three children under the age of five. She is depressed and finds she gets very irritable with her children. This is the reason given by the GP for the referral. She lives with a man who is younger than she is, who speaks little English, and is not the father of her children. Like Lisa, he is unemployed. They live in three rooms on the fourth floor and share a bathroom with other tenants. The children are frequent attendees at the GP surgery with minor ailments of one sort or another. Lisa has been previously treated with anti-depressants but this time has told the GP that she would prefer to talk to someone about her problems. On her patient's request form for counselling Lisa states that she would like weekly counselling over ten weeks (Service B).

Lisa fulfilled the counselling protocol requirements described in Chapter 3; she was motivated, there was a clear focus for work (her irritability with the children), she also recognized that her problems were at least in part psychological and she has explicitly chosen to work in words. With a referral like this, however, there may be a clear focus for work in the short term but there are also multiple long term problems which are situational and which cannot be helped very much by counselling (poverty, unemployment, housing, general deprivation). This is common in the patients referred for counselling help in an inner city practice.

Lisa needed support over time from various different parts of the flower diagram system (Fig. 3.1, Chapter 3) because her needs were great and the welfare of the young children was at stake. There was some degree of arbitrariness as to whether she should be referred by the GP to the complementary practitioners or to the counselling team. In fact, Lisa had earlier received massage, and it was when the four massage sessions were finished that the counselling referral was made. She had become ready to use words after becoming more reflective following the massage.

After her counselling sessions, she was able to see the relationship between her irritability with her children and these other pressures, particularly the pressure of feeling alone and child-like in the big city when she herself was a parent. Like her partner in a way, she had been unable to understand the 'language' of the city: where to get reliable support, where to learn how to manage her depression about being a child-parent, how to move from feeling alienated towards more of a sense of belonging. After some counselling, she was ready to accept a referral to the Community Mental Health Team (CMHT) for long term support, including practical help with managing her finances and with long term housing, whilst continuing to maintain her contact with the GP. This referral was facilitated by the practice counsellor, who undertook initial liaison with the CMHT.

Lisa's needs were first discussed 'in the round' in the primary health care team meeting attended by representatives of the CMHT as well as the health visitor and health centre clinicians. Because all members of the different professions and agencies continued to be in close touch (and, most importantly, Lisa knew this) she did not feel like a parcel sent from one destination to another but rather she was held and contained by a cooperative network. When she tried to divide the network and play one profession off against another, this pattern could be recognized, managed and contained and she could feel safe that she had not destroyed her care, as had happened in the past.

Clinically she was depressed, had interpersonal difficulties, stress, anxiety and underlying problems with loss and bereavement. Her multiple problems included housing, poverty, poor education and social isolation. Acting as members of a multi-professional and multi-agency team, from considering the referral to the completion of each individual piece of work, the GP, the massage therapist and then the counsellor helped her to access the different kinds of long term help she needed.

**Example – Sheila**   Counselling or complementary therapy?

Sheila is thirty eight and was referred to the counselling team by her GP because she has difficulty sleeping at night. The GP Referral Form indicates that Sheila also suffers from 'IBS' (irritable bowel syndrome). Her file shows that she works as a cleaner, and is married to the porter and caretaker of a block of flats. They live in two tiny rooms at the top of the old mansion block for which they are jointly responsible. They have no children and do not want any. Sheila has told her GP that she does not want to take sleeping tablets, but says it is difficult to be up at night when her husband has to go to work early as he gets cross about being woken up.

Sheila fills in the form for counselling, asking for one or two counselling sessions only (Service A). At the first assessment session, the counsellor suggests that she increase this to ten sessions (Service B) and Sheila at first agrees. During the early sessions her deeply unhappy and isolated life unfolds, but she decides that it is too painful to have more counselling and that she prefers to carry on with her life as it is. She says that she has never talked to anyone in this way before and does not want to go on and talk about sex, because she is sure that is where things are leading. The counsellor had not mentioned any such link.

Her main worry, Sheila explains, is that she will pass wind at night if she goes to sleep, and that this will make a smell which she finds embarrassing in their tiny flat, especially as her husband complains and calls her 'smelly' and 'windbag' if she does so. The counselling led her close to the relation between her worries about her bowels, her worries about sex, and her tight but precarious emotional control, and she decides to keep things as they are rather than to go deeper. Thus her choice of Service A, assessment only, is eventually borne out by the limits of her tolerance of internal change.

In this instance it would have been just as reasonable for the GP to have referred Sheila first to the naturopath, who could have scrutinized her diet and suggested suitable supplements or food combinations, or indeed to the massage therapist, who would have helped her to relax and taught her some breathing skills that would have helped her calm down before going to bed at night. Instead she saw the counsellor first, who then referred her for one assessment session to the naturopath. Again, Sheila decided to ignore most of the dietary advice she was given by him, preferring to continue buying dietary products from her favourite chemist as before.

It was important for Sheila to be offered both counselling and dietary advice, but it was also important that her eventual wish to protect the long term equilibrium in her life be recognized, when the implications of further counselling became clear to her. She went away with a deeper understanding of her difficulty in sleeping and her bowel problems, and a recognition that any inner change would be fairly disruptive to her security.

It emerged in the six sessions she attended, that her marriage had previously been very turbulent and her husband (who was very big and strong) had threatened once to throw her off the roof of the flats, had then climbed on to the roof himself after taking an overdose, and was admitted to hospital overnight. Sheila remembered too much of this sort of fear from her childhood in Ireland, which she had tried to put behind her. Like many patients, she was paying a price for their stability now, but was prepared to go on doing so rather than face further crises.

**Example – Hassan**   Redundancy

Hassan is forty five and has recently been made redundant from his job as an accountant in a large company. He has been unable to tell his wife and still leaves the house every day as if he were going to work. He spends his time at the library, looking at vacancies and filling in job applications. He is very tense and feels a failure, especially as he has been unable to get an interview for any of the jobs for which he has applied. He also has serious backache and moves very stiffly. He asks for fortnightly fifty minute sessions over twenty weeks on the patient's request form (Service C) and explains at the assessment that this is because he does not think his problems 'will go away in ten weeks'. He is clinically depressed but does not want to take medication.

The counsellor sees Hassan fortnightly and arranges, after discussion with both GP and massage therapist, for him to have four massage sessions during which he can also be taught relaxation skills. Neither the patient nor any member of the team expects that these interventions will make fundamental changes, but it is likely that they can temporarily reduce his stress levels and prevent a bad situation from becoming worse, often an acceptable aim in general practice. When Hassan's counselling sessions are finished, he accepts an offer of half-hour follow-up sessions on an intermittent basis every six weeks, which allows him to be seen four times over a further six months (Service D). By this time he has become more resigned to his position, has started going to the swimming pool regularly with his son and has been able to tell his wife about his situation.

**Example – Zelda**   Terminal care

Zelda, forty four, suffers from a very malignant form of leukaemia. Her family are abroad and she returned to the UK for treatment at one of the local teaching hospitals. She was living alone and knew that she did not have long to live. She asked for half-hour counselling sessions every few weeks (Service D, intermittent) 'because time is precious to me and I know how to use it'. After the second session she accepted the counsellor's suggestion of a referral for four massage sessions. She continued her counselling sessions until she was unexpectedly told at the hospital, after tests, that she had a further remission from her illness and decided to go back to spend more time with her family. The referral to the counselling service was very much led by this patient, a highly intelligent woman who knew and understood precisely what the choices in her situation were. She wanted someone to talk to, and knew that she could return at any time for further sessions. That the counselling led to massage therapy was a bonus for her, enhanced by the knowledge that massage therapist, counsellor and GP were cooperating in her care.

**Example – John**   Bereavement

John, fifty eight, is a legal adviser in a well known firm. His wife has just died after a long struggle with breast cancer. He asks for one or two sessions only (Service A) 'because there is not a lot to say really, is there? It's just life.' He nevertheless accepts gratefully the counsellor's offer of a referral to the massage therapist for four sessions in parallel with the counselling sessions at the time when he is at his lowest ebb. Most of all, he wants no fuss and that he should be able to come to terms with his pain.

**Example – Mahmoud** Chronic pain and loneliness

Mahmoud, twenty seven, is an archivist in a local library. He has never made any intimate friendships and has no family in the UK. He lives alone in a bed-sit and suffers from sciatica, which sometimes keeps him off work. He was referred to the counselling team after he unexpectedly came close to tears when seeing a locum GP; he asked only for one or two sessions (Service A). Mahmoud kept the first counselling appointment, but cancelled the second on the day of the session and did not recontact the counselling team after the 'nudge' letter. When he next saw another GP she referred him to the osteopath, after which he recontacted the counsellor on his own initiative and arranged four more sessions. During this time it became clear that he was very seriously disturbed, and that further uncovering work was contraindicated because it could lead to his breakdown. This risk was discussed between counsellor and patient, and he decided to return to the GP to get some medication to help him cope with a life that was always going to be difficult.

**Example – Leila** Transition from physical pain to mental pain

Leila, fifty eight, is well known to the GPs for her chronic indigestion and bowel problems. She is a large, well dressed and made-up woman who wears a great deal of jewellery and elaborate, expensive clothes when she comes to the surgery. She often goes to see private doctors in nearby Harley Street if she cannot get what she wants from the centre. She has so far resisted all attempts by her woman GP to talk about her home life, but one day opens up with a story about her husband and his mistresses. She becomes very tearful and accepts a counselling referral. She fills in her Patient's Request Form asking for brief work (Service B). The counselling sessions reveal a family trauma, which took place some twenty years before, in which her sister, brother and mother were drowned in front of her. She was the only survivor.

Counselling made little difference to her mental or physical symptoms, however. She seemed just to like coming to the surgery to talk, almost as if it were a social occasion, even about such a serious trauma. The GP noticed, however, that after the ten counselling sessions she was easier to communicate with and exerted less pressure for new solutions. Leila then agreed to an appointment with the naturopath who advised her on certain aspects of her diet and prescribed some dietary supplements. After this, Leila arranged another appointment with the counsellor just to thank her for all she had made possible. The story will continue, but somehow there is a feeling that this patient has begun to understand the relationship between her mind and her body a little more and will put less pressure on the professionals for magical solutions.

## ASSESSMENT

Assessment was briefly referred to when considering the audit context of referrals above. It is a major topic, about which much has been written, and can be a major part of brief counselling work whatever the setting. Burton considers it the vital issue, not only for the training and supervision of counsellors, but also if meaningful evaluation is to be conducted. She pro-

> **Figure 4.3**   Purposes of counselling assessment sessions at Marylebone Health Centre
>
> - to explore the patient's expectations and hopes of counselling
> - to clarify what counselling can or cannot offer and whether this 'fits'
> - to establish the limits and boundaries (time, place, confidentiality within the team etc.)
> - to clarify the focus for counselling
> - to test out the patient's response to some preliminary forays at understanding
> - to review the choice of counselling service in the light of need and expectations (Services A–F)
> - to discuss the £5 contribution per session (unless the patient is unwaged)
> - to exclude patients who are unsuitable for counselling, commonly patients who
>   - are conspicuous consumers of care services
>   - have strong somatic elements to their presentation
>   - are too fragile
>   - are either already receiving community psychiatric services or clearly need to do so
>   - are already in some form of counselling or psychotherapy elsewhere or in complementary therapy at Marylebone

vides a detailed discussion of the various assessment instruments available to counsellors in primary care (Burton 1998). However, for very brief work of approximately twelve sessions, assessment can consume resources disproportionately in relation to the counselling work itself. Somehow, rightly or wrongly, this is not the case at Marylebone.

Partly, this is because we assume that in the inner city we are going to be faced with complex internal and external problems of a bio-psycho-social nature. We are also fortunate to be part of a containing network of professionals who take a pragmatic approach and work fairly closely together. Every session is seen as a form of continuing assessment, carried out in partnership with the patient. In addition the GP referral form, the patient request form and the menu of counselling services enable us carefully to manage key aspects of assessment. The motivation test of the patient request form has addressed one aspect satisfactorily: patients who do not demonstrate their motivation by completing the form are now simply not offered an appointment (emergencies aside) and almost one third of our clinical time has been saved as a result.

Having established that there is some degree of motivation, the next question is for what? Often patients have no idea that counselling can be a disturbing experience. Sheila, in the above example, illustrates this point clearly. The patient's choice of counselling service is therefore only a limited indicator of what type of help is being sought, although it helps when discussing the framework of patients' expectations and wishes. For this reason the first one or two assessment sessions are used by the counsellor in the ways listed in Figure 4.3.

The assessments of Sheila, Leila and Lisa, and to some extent Hassan and Mahmoud, in reality continued beyond the first session or two into the brief work itself. Each had a focus for work at the start, which we continued to refine and explore as the work continued. We thus begin by accepting the patient's definition of the problem, which has already been developed a little in the preparatory sessions with the GP. Then, we continue to refine the focus with the patient's help, as the work progresses.

Thus, for example, it could be gradually recognized by counsellor and patient that Mahmoud was being made more fragile by counselling, which was not the best solution for him. Similarly with Lisa, patient and counsellor could bring her situational needs into sharper focus, and see how they made her more irritable with the children, and then work on setting up a long term support network. With Leila, there was some tough negotiation about her relationship with the health centre, and although it seemed initially that she needed to work through her newly-revealed 'survivor guilt', this turned out not to be the case after all. The counselling episode was just one chapter in a long saga of care, and perhaps the referral was inappropriate or the assessment should have picked up that counselling was not likely to help. That would have been a difficult decision to make in one session however, and one could equally argue that, given that the work was only going to be brief, it was appropriate to give her the benefit of the doubt. The GPs were helped by the small temporary changes that they noticed in how Leila used their services whilst she was seeing the counsellor, which provided justification in terms of 'sharing the load'. Sheila, on the other hand, who was seen before the menu of services was fully in place, used her counselling sessions to arrive at a greater understanding of her problems, only to decide that enough was enough. In such brief work one has sometimes to assess quickly the limits of what is possible, and to recognize that fragile equilibrium in the inner city can be better that no equilibrium at all.

These examples of referral and assessment can best be summarized as a pragmatic and patient-centred approach, with modest aims, in a context of inter-professional teamwork with the GPs and complementary therapists, and inter-agency work with other community agencies.

In the counselling team, we draw on our range of different skills and experience: psychodynamic and cognitive, stress management, crisis intervention and psycho-social. Each assessment is usually discussed in supervision, where the counselling focus is scrutinized and often refined, and the resource allocation is reviewed. Where a patient is in very great need, we will discuss this immediately after the first session. For example, where a refugee has been tortured (as in Chapter 12), or a patient has a long term mental health problem (as in Chapter 9), it is necessary to consider whether to make an outside referral for further work, or whether it is more appropriate to discuss the long term need with the patient and to earmark an intermittent service slot (Service D). In all brief work the end is in sight at the beginning, and it is necessary to face the implications with the patient and within supervision at that point.

## Supervision

In the assessment supervision session we try to arrive at a summary based on the work of Malan (1979) which links the focus of a current life problem (C for current) with the 'here and now' of interaction with the counsellor (T for transference) and, if it is known, the past life (P for past). This TCP framework, described by Malan as the 'triangle of insight', provides a means of refining and continuing to supervise the focus. It has been shown to be linked to effective outcomes and is extremely useful for supervisor and counsellor as a guide to where to look, when to interpret or what is missing in the material so far. It is not always possible, however, to complete a full triangular formulation of this kind in very brief work, usually because some material has not been forthcoming, or the counsellor is not yet clear how s/he is being used in the transference or 'here and now'.

Sometimes it is not desirable to follow such a framework because the patient brings a working framework of his/her own as with Zelda and John, both of whom were coping in their own ways with different aspects of bereavement and its impact on life as they knew it. It would have been inappropriate and artificial to modify or extend their formulations of why they were attending counselling. It was much more appropriate for them to be provided with time, a place and the person of the counsellor to use in the way that they defined and needed.

Individual supervision at Marylebone has only recently been reduced to once a month for one and a half hours in line with the recommended minimum of the British Association of Counsellors. This is preferable to fifty minutes or one hour, because it allows more than one case to be discussed. It also provides some room for discussing audit and management of the counselling system, and the context of changing policies of the health centre and of primary care locally and nationally.

At different phases in the development of each counsellor receiving supervision, the approach taken is varied to meet their needs. For example, at induction, the four counsellors in the Counselling Volunteer and Supervison Scheme felt overwhelmed by the context, and it was important that they became oriented to the setting before seeing patients. Each observed at least one GP surgery in full, and one hour of a busy period of work by the receptionists. They wrote up their accounts of these observations and of their own reactions and then brought these for discussion in supervision. These sessions allowed the nature of the problems brought to a busy inner city practice to be understood, the counsellors' individual preconceptions about GPs and general practice to be examined, and the pressures on different parts of the multi-professional team to be recognized.

The next phase involved discussing in detail the first assessment sessions and early work undertaken, particularly with regard to identifying and maintaining a focus, excluding inappropriate patients, managing counselling resources through the Menu of Services and record keeping. Next to be discussed were issues around managing diaries in relation to the different services and to ending, with most counsellors finding this aspect difficult as neither counselling nor psychotherapy training sufficiently equips them for setting clinical priorities in a context where demands are so rapid and so varied, or for such brief work.

As counsellors become more accustomed to the rhythms of very brief work, it is easier to use supervision to focus more on clinical depth and precision and to plan ahead. The instrument we use first for clinical supervision is process recording. The counsellors are asked to write a detailed account of their own and the patient's interactions, from the point of receiving the referral and reading the file to the session itself, and their reflections after the session is finished. The notes should include feelings, fears, uncertainties, blunders and, within limits, the counsellor's own associations with the material. Some counsellors find this detail difficult, depending on what kind of supervision they have previously received, and a clear boundary needs to be kept between the counsellor's own psychotherapy or counselling and the supervision task.

At first, some counsellors may not see the relevance of process recordings, but the use of such material, first as a vehicle for understanding processes of interaction and next for some straight teaching, usually enables the work to proceed. Clinical notes should also be scrutinized regularly, to ensure appropriate recording is taking place and that important aspects of a patient's history or current treatment are sufficiently considered. If, as can happen, a counsellor refuses to expose his/her work in this way, or does not accept the authority of supervisor or GP, it is necessary for the supervisor to explain carefully the interdependent nature of teamwork in the setting. It may eventually be necessary to give an official warning, in discussion with and supported by the GP, pointing out the system of clinical accountability. In such a situation, the notes kept by the supervisor on the initial framework agreed for supervision, and to which counsellor and supervisor are both accountable, are invaluable. These notes should be clear and can be used as a reference point for resolving problems within the agreed framework. Notes kept on each individual supervision session are also used, at Marylebone, as a way of monitoring how work with each patient progresses and how resources are used. They also provide material for periodic reviews of the development needs of the counsellor and the usefulness of the supervision, including areas of development for the supervisor.

Initially however, the emotional impact of the kind of stressful work described in Chapter 1 is considerable and it is important for supervision to provide sufficient time for digesting this impact and then normalizing it. Over-professionalization, in the form of too much distance or 'too thick a skin', needs to be avoided in what is, after all, a frontline setting. When new counsellors join the team at Marylebone, supervision is offered on a weekly basis during the four-week induction period, and then becomes fortnightly. The whole counselling team meets every other month for a three-way case discussion of one and a half hours, to allow experience to be discussed 'in the round' instead of in the line management system, and for a period an experienced counsellor from another practice joined this discussion, a practice which we recommend as bearing fruit for all.

## COUNSELLING RECORDS AND CONFIDENTIALITY

Confidentiality and counselling records are linked issues and are somewhat controversial areas. It is common for counsellors in general practice to keep their records separately from the GPs and other members of the primary health care team. Confidentiality in that model of record-keeping is usually taken to mean 'confidentiality between the counsellor and patient'. A good discussion of the issues involved can be found in Rain (1997), who distinguishes between records kept for supervision, those placed in the patient's health record file, and longer records of assessments and final summaries; in effect, three different types of records. Even so, Rain makes it clear that records belong to the practice, and ultimately to the health authority, not to the counsellor. Other key publications convey how contested these issues are in the field.

Sibbald et al, on behalf of the RCGP (1996a), warn that communication can become imperilled if practice counsellors refuse to divulge any information about patients' progress in counselling to third parties such as GPs. They suggest that because counselling training is in a more individualistic tradition than the teamwork approach of general practice, it is difficult for counsellors to adapt to information sharing. They conclude that where counsellors refuse to share information both in records and discussion, a model of working results which is 'alien to general practitioners and possibly unworkable in general practice' (p. 16). They also consider that 'matters of referral, information exchange, and patient confidentiality are central to the development of counselling services within general practice' (p16).

The British Association of Counsellors: Counselling in Medical Settings Section (BACCMS) guidelines, published before Sibbald's work, indicate that maintaining appropriate patient records, including audit and an annual report, should be part of the job description of counsellors in general practice (BAC 1993). However, the view put forward here differs significantly from both Rain (1997) and Sibbald et al (1996a) in stating categorically that counsellors records 'should be separate from the medical notes and kept in a locked drawer to maintain confidentiality. Any information recorded in the medical notes should be agreed with the client' (p. 6, Section 4). The BACCMS also refers to the fact that, since the Access to Health Records Act 1991, patients can have access to their records, although whether they consider the counsellor's locked away records should be subject to this legislation is not clear.

At Marylebone Health Centre we do not keep separate records or files for counselling (other than the process recordings used in supervision), because we believe that by compartmentalizing information (and hence understanding) we would undermine the whole person approach the practice seeks to maintain. We write brief notes in the patient's medical records, in chronological order with those of the GP and other health care professionals, such as the health visitor, practice or district nurse or complementary therapist. The narrative of professional interventions in the patient's life history is therefore integrated to tell a unified and continuing story. We explain to the patient at the beginning verbally, and in the counselling leaflet, that the confidentiality boundary is with the health centre team and not with the individual counsellor. Patients often come to Marylebone Health Centre because they know of its whole person approach and teamwork, and they understand that collaboration and information sharing is essential.

Separate records can foster a kind of unhealthy splitting between the counsellor and the GP, which is often to the patients' disadvantage and may be unwittingly exploited by them, in the process feeding into latent rivalries. Inevitably, counsellors provide more time (thirty to fifty mins) for the patient as against the GP's ten minutes. The counsellor sees, on average, four to five patients in an afternoon, whereas the GP may see as many as twenty five. It is thus easy for the patient to see the GP as the busy one 'who does not listen' and the counsellor as a special kind of listener; conversely, the GP may be seen as the nice, down-to-earth, practical one, whilst the counsellor's focus on feelings may be felt to be at once too threatening and not practical enough. In fact, GP and counsellor are members of the same team and, although their expertise and perspectives differ, they share a common concern for the patient.

The counselling records are brief and to the point, and written in such a way that should the patient, as is now legally permitted, request to see them, what is read will contain no surprises in the form of hidden professional or clinical judgements; rather, the notes record the essence of what has been said in the counselling session, using as far as possible the same words that patient and counsellor have used. Some typical examples drawn from the case studies outlined above now follow.

Record 1 gives the GP slightly more information than before and casts a new light on the limited choices before Lisa. It allows some thinking to

---

**Record 1:** Lisa

Session 2: Lisa explained problems with children, particularly Kevin, four, who provokes partner, Mahmoud, by shouting English words at him and running away. She feels caught between them and wishes that M would find somewhere else to live but 'feels sorry for him'. They met in the pub four months ago and have been together since. I took up Lisa's isolation with three small children under five, and her own feelings of being a child in the big city without helpful adult company. Also asked about her past. Father of the children (Johnny) now in prison, used to beat her and children. 'At least things are better without him.' Next session: Wed 6th Dec 3.00 p.m.

---

**Record 2:** Kevin

Kevin is said by his mother to have difficulties with her new partner Mahmoud who does not speak English: K is said to shout English words at him. Sounds distressed and angry at losing his own father, Johnny (in prison), and having to share his depressed mother with several others. Will need careful assessment if brought with a minor ailment. (Information from mother's counselling session.)

---

**Record 3:** Leila

Session 2: Leila wanted to use counselling to discuss physical symptoms. I pointed out that she had asked for counselling because she thought, like the GP, that these symptoms were caused by unhappiness. 'I am not an unhappy person. I try always to be cheerful.' Pause – then tears. 'My husband does not love me any more. He always has young girls. I try to look good. One day I shall get an infection. My life is over. It was over a long time ago.' There followed a story of the death by drowning of her original family, with herself the only survivor looking on. She has never forgiven herself, nor the ferryboat owners who had failed to maintain the boat on which the family died. Next session: Fri Nov 4th 4.00 p.m.

---

**Record 4:** Hassan

Session 1: Hassan came in a suit with briefcase. Very formal and polite. Showed me his job application file. I commented on the major change from being a busy, respected professional to having to start again with nothing yet in sight. 'The problem is I have this backache. It stops me doing lots of things. I would like to do a lot more. To go and see people, sell myself and all that.' I said it must be difficult to go and sell himself when perhaps he was feeling unsure about what there was to sell at present. Said he does not expect much change in short term but wants counselling sessions as he has no-one to talk to. He has not told his wife yet. I suggested a parallel referral for massage which he welcomed. Next session: fortnight today.

---

take place about the need for good long term support within the inter-agency network. A further note is made on the child Kevin's file by the counsellor.

An example of the risks in shared notes in the medical record now follows.

---

**Record 5:** Tamara

---

Session 5: Worrying session. Tamara talked of her despair and suicidal thoughts. Had bought a large bottle of paracetamol and some whisky 'for the cupboard'. I said she clearly wanted me to take the worry seriously and knew that the GP would do so as well. Is moving from address to address so one never quite knows if she is going to turn up. Discussed suicidal risk in supervision and with Dr Brown.

---

The next week this patient came in to see a new practice nurse to complete a life insurance form for the GP to sign. The nurse noted the comments about suicidal risk on the GP referral form and in the notes, but did not ask the patient why she was taking out a life insurance at this time, and did not tell the counsellor about the request. She included the information about the suicidal risk on the form, and the GP signed it and the insurance was refused. The patient was furious. There followed much debate about the wisdom of shared records, about the procedures for completing life insurance forms and about vehicles for team communication between part-time staff; the failure of communication between different members of the team was also discussed. The fact is that the patient is in no doubt that her suicidal ideas have been taken seriously by the practice, and that she can have help from the GP and counsellor if she wants it.

These brief notes thus provide an aide-memoire to the counsellor, and a vehicle of communication between the counsellor, the GP and other clinical staff who have little weekly time to discuss the work, and may not even be at the practice on the same day. After every counselling session, the patient's notes are placed in the GP's tray to indicate that a session has taken place and to update the GP. Similarly, when the counsellor sees the patient, the notes are put out ready before the session by the receptionist, so that any other contacts the patient has made with the practice since the last counselling appointment can be noted.

At Marylebone we believe that communication by records is a vital part of counselling in general practice, where the patient may well see other members of the team, particularly the GP, between the counselling sessions. It is also in line with Jenifer Elton Wilson's critique of some counsellors' attitudes, when she points out that counselling is not necessarily the central influence on a patient's life and development, but is part of a complex web of influences (Elton Wilson 1996, p. 5).

## CLINICAL AND MANAGERIAL RESPONSIBILITY

Two of the reasons given in the literature for good, shared records are that the GP carries final clinical responsibility for what happens in the event, for example, of a suicide, and that counsellors rarely have a sound enough training in mental health or psychopathology to carry full clinical responsibility. This issue of clinical responsibility, and the linked issue of malpractice insurance, is beginning to be debated more openly with regard to counselling in general practice. However, because a number of different models of employment and clinical responsibility are in use in the field, it is a debate which is difficult to focus, since the issues change somewhat according to the context. We will therefore confine our remarks to our own context.

At Marylebone Health Centre the issue of responsibility, whether clinical or managerial, rests finally with one of the principal GPs. She is responsible in turn to the GP partners and the multi-professional practice management group, which includes all of the GP team, the practice manager and managers of the part-time clinical units. This means that if there were a dispute between a counsellor and a GP, or if a patient believed that malpractice had occurred, the GP and hence his/her insurer, the Medical Defence Union or the Medical Protection Society, would respond to the complaint and would carry ultimate authority and responsibility.

Clinical and managerial responsibility are therefore united in one person (the GP) and one structure (medical responsibility). Although for some counsellors this may seem an odd arrangement, for psychotherapists it is a common one. Indeed, some psychotherapy organizations (such as several of the constituent members of the British Confederation of Psychotherapists) require that both medical cover and medical responsibility arrangements are made and are explicit as a condition of membership.

The issue of clinical responsibility is never as straightforward as it would appear, however. The assumption that finally the GPs are clinically responsible does not mean that counsellors are not. It is desirable that counsellors should feel fully responsible and accountable for their clinical work, and not be tempted to hide behind the medical responsibility that is part and parcel of a medical setting. Although our system has yet to be tried in terms of a counselling complaint, counsellors at the centre are required to carry their own independent malpractice insurance, in addition to that of the GPs. In any claim, the counsellor will in any event be held responsible for his/her work in its own right, whilst the GP will be held professionally responsible for vetting the qualifications and competence of the counsellor to practice, and for establishing appropriate communication, monitoring and records practices. There is a tension here, and a necessary one, between the clinical and managerial responsibility for the whole of the work of the multi-professional team, which lies with the GP and extends to cover all aspects of clinical practice carried out at the GP's request, and the individual clinical responsibility of the counsellor for his own professional practice. This tension is a safeguard for the patient because it ensures that two-way accountability exists between counsellor and GP.

## IN CONCLUSION ...

It is easy for the multi-professional approach of Marylebone to be seen as generous, although the reality is that services are strictly limited and time-conscious. The issue of doubling-up on counselling and complementary therapy services is scrutinized carefully to avoid conspicuous consumers of services and target the extended range of care and treatment services to those in greatest need. Referral, audit, assessment, supervision, record-keeping and clinical responsibility are, as Sibbald and her colleagues stated (1996a), central to the business of counselling in general practice, and the issues are complex. At Marylebone, we have resolved these complexities in our own way, but our resolution is constantly and necessarily under review because there are no easy solutions.

# 5

# A profile of one year's counselling: improvisation and routine

*Alison Vaspe*

Listening to one another and to themselves, [reflective practitioners] feel where the music is going and adjust their playing accordingly. They are inventing on-line, and they are also responding to surprises provided by the inventions of others[...]

Donald Schön, 'The crisis of professional knowledge and the pursuit of an epistemology of practice' *Journal of Interprofessional Care*

---

## SYNOPSIS

This chapter draws upon the ten years of experience of counselling at Marylebone to show the evolving picture of the counsellors' work. This profile of activity is set in the context of Marylebone's need for a well run resource, and of recent NHS policy changes which aim to make health services more accountable, effective and transparent in the way they are managed.

The various forms of audit undertaken by the counselling team are first described and then reviewed to present a profile of counselling referrals and patterns of work over a typical year. The Menu of Services described in Chapter 3 is then shown in action, illustrating its potential for disciplined but flexible management of limited counselling resources. Certain rhythms that are characteristic of general practice emerge. These are complex and lively. To give an idea of how practitioners work with them, Donald Schön's analogy with the performance of jazz is borrowed (Schön 1992). Just as jazz music involves a play on repeated elements ('routines') and improvisation, so the combination of the predictable and the random is at the heart of general practice.

---

## AUDITING THE COUNSELLORS' WORK

The counselling team currently reports on its activities by carrying out two forms of audit (Fig. 5.1).

- The practice and health authority audits require all members of the multi-professional team to fill in day sheets which are drawn up by recep-

---

**Figure 5.1**   Audit of the counsellors' work

- Practice and health authority audit: day sheets and practice database
  — numbers of patients seen
  — demographic details: age, sex, postal code, ethnicity
  — attendance patterns: kept appointments, lateness, cancellations, DNAs
- Counsellors' internal audit: GP Referral Form and Patient Request Form
  — employment status
  — waiting time between referral and first appointment
  — pattern of work: specific service (A–E) and number of sessions
  — presenting problems as seen by GP
  — outcome (medication and attendance rates pre- and post-counselling; referral to other agencies)

---

tion; these provide information on the number of patients seen and their attendance patterns. Patients' demographic details are available from the practice's computerized database.

- The counselling team carries out a separate audit using the GP referral form and patient request form. Together, these forms provide information about the pattern of work (Services A–E) chosen by patients and the problems leading to referral; outcome information on medication and attendance rates at the surgery pre- and post-counselling, and referral to other agencies have recently also been included.

In the year beginning January 1999 the counselling team, alongside some other practices making up the local Primary Care Group, will be taking part in a pilot of the Clinical Outcome in Routine Evaluation (CORE) system developed by the Psychological Therapies Research Centre at the University of Leeds (CORE System Group 1998). This centrally processed system makes the collection of data about clinical effectiveness part of routine practice. The approach is naturalistic and aims to generate large amounts of data from which guidelines setting standards of provision and treatment can be drawn up. A further important aim is to link practitioners and researchers in the service of evidence-based practice. The research tool consists of:

- an outcome measure completed by the patient and addressing the clinical domains of subjective well-being, symptoms, functioning and risk/harm
- an evaluative audit tool completed by the practitioner at two points of patient contact: assessment and end of episode
- further components of the system which are currently being developed include
  — a service and provider profile
  — an idiographic tool for measuring patient goals and their subsequent attainment

— a measure for assessing the working alliance.

This chapter will however draw upon existing audit data from the ten years of counselling at Marylebone in order to give both a picture of the evolving system and a profile of a typical year's activity at this point in time.

## THE PROFILE OF A YEAR'S COUNSELLING

### Numbers of patients referred for counselling and patterns of work

The following discussion assumes the availability of three counsellors providing approximately ten hours (three three and a half hour sessions) per week for forty seven weeks per year.

Over the years the counselling service has been in action the number of counselling referrals made per year has remained fairly constant: approximately thirty five patients per year per three and a half hour counselling session. This figure is largely determined by GPs' awareness of the availability of counselling and the length of the waiting list at any one time. The development of Patient Request Forms has, however, resulted in around 25% of referrals discontinuing at the point of GP referral, with no waste of counselling session or administration time. This means an average of eighty one patients now attend for counselling each year.

Furthermore, changes in the number of counselling sessions taken up by patients as a result of developing the Menu of Counselling Services, and in particular Service A (one or two exploratory sessions) and Service D, will allow a greater number of patients to be referred for counselling over the year and, equally as important, to be contained by the team at any one point in time. Figure 5.2 shows how, over the year, one counsellor, working

**Figure 5.2** Developing the Menu of Counselling Services: notional profile of one counsellor's caseload over one year

| Service | No. Patients |
| --- | --- |
| A (1 or 2 exploratory sessions only) | 9 |
| B (weekly sessions of 50 minutes for about 10 weeks) | 6 |
| C (fortnightly sessions of 50 minutes for about 20 weeks) | 6 |
| D (intermittent 30- or 50-minute sessions every 4–6 weeks over a longer period) | 7 |
| E (up to 10 weekly or fortnightly sessions of 30 minutes) | 3 |
| X (1 emergency session plus follow-up) | 2 |
| Total | 33 |

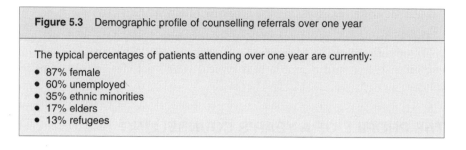

**Figure 5.3** Demographic profile of counselling referrals over one year

The typical percentages of patients attending over one year are currently:

- 87% female
- 60% unemployed
- 35% ethnic minorities
- 17% elders
- 13% refugees

for one three and a half hour session per week, can now carry thirty three patients working for different periods, from one or two sessions only (Service A) to around 30 sessions over a period of four years (Service D). Taking into account the 25% of DNAs at first session before the referral process was tightened, the service has therefore seen an increase in the numbers of patients actually seen from under seventy, to eighty one, to a potential figure of nearly one hundred.

## Demographic profile and presenting problems of counselling referrals

Figure 5.3 shows the current demographic profile of counselling referrals over a typical year. Marylebone's open door policy towards patient registration, which is skewed to those with limited finances and in greater need (see Chapter 2), is reflected in the number of unwaged patients who, either because they are students or pensioners, or because of unemployment, now make up nearly two-thirds of counselling referrals.

Three important groups of patients have in the past been identified as under-represented in counselling referrals at Marylebone:

- young adults (under twenty years)
- elders (sixty five years or over)
- ethnic minorities.

While the provision of student counselling services in local higher education establishments largely accounts for the low rate of referrals of under-twenties to the counsellors, cultural assumptions about elders and ethnic minorities were discussed in the multi-professional team as a reason for their under-representation as a group of referrals.

Elders may be referred in lower numbers because of decreased mobility, which means that GPs and district nurses provide the bulk of their care. However, their greater emotional strength and self-reliance, as well as the sense of time running out, has been shown to be a motivating factor and to lead to their making good use of brief counselling (Terry 1997).

For ethnic minorities, ignorance of other cultures as well as prejudice, have been identified as factors leading not just to their under-representation in counselling and psychology services, but also to their over-representation in psychiatric diagnoses of mental disturbance (Fernando 1995).

Highlighting underlying assumptions about the suitability of these groups of people for counselling has led to substantial changes, especially in the number of referrals from ethnic minorities, which now account for over a third of all referrals. Furthermore, some 'Caucasian' patients are from overseas, and include refugees from war-torn countries. Refugees as a group now represent a significant proportion of counselling referrals: 13% of the total as compared to under 2% in 1989–1990 (Webber et al 1996). The severity of their problems on all levels – physical, practical and emotional – has an impact on the whole practice team.

As is typically the case in counselling services, a large number of referrals are women, at something under 90%. The majority of these are in the twenty to thirty five age group, followed by those in the thirty six to fifty age group. This probably says something about women's greater ability to articulate their feelings, their expectation that talking about problems will be helpful, and also about social expectations that feelings are a woman's problem.

The presenting problems of counselling referrals reflect changing social attitudes. In 1989–1990 the counselling service at Marylebone broke down primary and secondary reasons for referral into eight problem areas (Webber et al 1996):

- alcoholism
- bereavement
- depression
- financial problem
- housing problem
- refugee issue
- relationship problem
- general stress.

The largest numbers of referrals were for relationship problems, general stress, depression and difficulties around life transitions, and relationship break-up or loss due to unemployment or bereavement (see Chapter 3).

Definition of a patient's problem was often made by the referring GP and confirmed by the counsellor following assessment. Since then, these descriptors have been changed and developed as a result of the local health authority's request for additional categories, particularly with a view to identifying a patient's psychological state at presentation. The current system (Fig. 5.4) categorizes patients' presentations for counselling under two broad headings: 'internal' and 'external' problems, or psychological/ emotional state and life events. The headings are not mutually exclusive but aim to give a rounded picture of patients' problems.

**Figure 5.4**   Patients' problem categories

- Internal (state of mind)
  — depression
  — anxiety
  — panic attack/performance anxiety
  — stress
  — parasuicidal
  — severe mental illness
  — psychosomatic
  — eating disorder
  — self-harm/victim tendency
  — addiction problems
  — compulsive behaviour
  — violence
- External (life events)
  — bereavement/loss
  — relationship difficulties
  — sexual problems
  — fertility problems
  — unemployment/redundancy
  — abuse/post-abuse
  — post traumatic stress disorder (PTSD)/victim of crime
  — serious physical illness or injury
  — transitions
  — refugee/displaced person
  — financial difficulties
  — housing problems
  — domestic violence
  — harassment
  — carer/dependant issues
  — problems relating to study/work

The change in categorizing patients' problems makes comparison over the years difficult. Furthermore, the policy of the counselling team in recent years has altered the profile of counselling referrals. The counsellors' switch to a commitment to the care culture now means that they see a significant number of patients suffering from complex problems, sometimes involving multi-professional and/or inter-agency collaboration. These include mental health problems, chronic physical illness, domestic violence, and work with refugees. One measure of the level of distress or disturbance in Marylebone patients referred for counselling may be found in the statistic that the percentage in whom depression was a feature on presentation has risen from under 10% in 1989–1990 to a little under 75% in 1997–1998.

On the one hand, the new policy could be criticized for over-inclusion. On the other, it reflects a deepening understanding in the counselling team of the kind of service needed in inner city general practice, where the problems of shifting populations, rootlessness and job insecurity impact upon individuals in harsh and sudden ways that can precipitate emotional crises and destabilize otherwise uneventful lives.

## RESPONSE TIMES AND PATTERNS OF WORK

A substantial literature has demonstrated that a prompt response to a patient's request for counselling is one of the key factors in satisfactory outcomes. Our performance target at Marylebone is for an appointment letter to be sent out within two weeks or, if that is not possible, a letter asking the patient if he or she wishes to be placed on a waiting list. Seen in relation to waiting times for longer term counselling and psychotherapy in the NHS, two weeks may seem no time at all. However, in general practice expectations are different. Patients may be in the middle of a life event, including serious illness or following a suicide attempt, and the need to talk about their experiences is often urgent. Left too long, some revert to habitual coping patterns or find the pain and difficulty of re-opening their emotional wounds too much when weighed against the as yet unknown benefits of counselling.

The gate-opening skills of the GPs depend upon a knowledge of the number and nature of counselling hours available, as well as what the counsellors can and cannot do for their patients. Their increasingly sophisticated knowledge helps ensure that, though waiting lists may at times be inevitable, they remain on the whole fairly manageable. The knock-on benefit is that most referrals do come through to their first appointment successfully, and that the presentations to the counsellor are not distorted too much by feelings about having to wait. This awareness of the counsellors' capacities is the key to the successful running of an integrated service, so an absolute priority of the counsellors, however busy they may be, is to keep the GPs in touch with their workload by circulating monthly progress reports.

The increasing number of patients who opt for Service A and Service D has been noted. At one end of the time-scale, the exploratory sessions of Service A allow patients one or two fifty minute sessions (five times the length of a regular GP appointment) to gain some insight into their problems or life situation. Occasionally, a choice is made to continue working over a longer period. Often, however, the counsellors have found that a tick in the Service A box means a patient wants just that. At the other extreme, the intermittent (every four to six weeks) sessions of Service D provide patients with a long term supportive relationship and a regular thinking space that can help them cope with severe and ongoing problems such as psychiatric conditions, terminal illness, or long term family or work difficulties. Providing this service also gives the counsellors a valued experience of long term relationships with patients, and hence allows a closer connection to be made to the work of GPs and nurses, who also get to know their patients over years rather than months.

## THE RHYTHMS OF THE GENERAL PRACTICE YEAR: IMPROVISATION AND ROUTINE

The rhythms of general practice are complex and quick. Counsellors coming into this setting can find themselves baffled and wrong-footed by the pace set by those around them, who are trained and used to working in small spaces under constant pressure. The pace has quickened and become yet more complex over recent years as a result of NHS policy changes (see Chapter 6). These changes have demanded flexibility and rapid assimilation of information, as well as new working patterns, from all in the general practice team. The art of being a counsellor in this context sometimes seems to lie in a combination of improvisation in response to these rhythms, and the ability to protect the quiet spaces and slower pacing needed for the counselling work itself.

### An annual cycle of counselling referrals

Rates of counselling referrals are always to some extent random and unpredictable but some patterns do recur from year to year. Referrals tend to peak, for example, at times of festival or holiday when those with families prepare to spend time with them, while those without those ties may feel a painful sense of lack.

Figure 5.5 shows the typical pattern of referral over one year. As ethnic minority referrals increase, peak times for counselling can be seen to occur

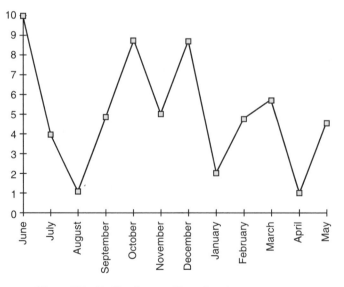

**Figure 5.5**   Profile of counselling referrals over one year

before holiday periods and the main Christian, Jewish and Hindu religious festivals in:

- June (the start of the long months of summer)
- early autumn
  - two key Hindu festivals, Diwali (the Festival of Light), closely followed by the New Year
  - two key Jewish festivals, New Year (Rosh Hashana), followed by the Day of Atonement (Yom Kippur)
- December (Christmas)
- and, to a lesser extent, March (Easter; Jewish Passover).

The Muslim year is based on a lunar calendar which is six days shorter than the calendar in general use in this country. This means that Ramadan, a key religious festival involving a thirty day period of fasting during daylight hours, may over time fall during the long days of summer or the shorter days of winter.

## Meetings

Against the fluctuations of referral highs and lows, the fixed points of team and network meetings provide a steady beat, and generate a counter rhythm of demand and expectations. These practice meetings have been described in detail in Chapter 2. Figure 5.6 shows them in profile over one year.

Donald Schön observes that,

the collective process of musical invention is not usually undertaken at random ... It is organized around an underlying structure – a shared scheme of meter, melody and harmony that gives the piece a predictable order. In addition, each of the musicians has a repertoire of musical figures that he can play, weaving variations of them as the opportunity arises. Improvisation consists in varying, combining and recombining a set of figures within the scheme that gives coherence to the whole performance (Schön 1992, p. 59)

For the counsellors at Marylebone, this structure is made up of the different patterns of work in the menu of counselling services, and the regular meetings with the counselling team, the multi-professional team, and the inter-agency network.

Against the long beats of the four-monthly review meetings, culminating in the summer AGM for which a full report is prepared, the rotating Wednesday lunchtime meetings allow a regular space for the problems and processes of the multi-professional team and inter-agency network to be heard. Within the counselling team, a combination of monthly supervision and six-weekly case discussion meetings act as an internal sounding board for the team to listen to each other and to feel heard by colleagues who share the stresses and strains of the counselling year.

**Figure 5.6** Profile of counsellors' team and network meetings over one year

| Week (Jan–Dec) | Wednesday lunchtime meetings | Counsellors and counsellor/GP meetings | Other meetings with counsellor representation |
|---|---|---|---|
| 1 | Primary health care | | |
| 2 | Process | Supervision | Practice management |
| 3 | Academic | Case discussion | |
| 4 | Staff | Collaborative task | Practice management |
| 5 | Primary health care | | |
| 6 | Process | Supervision | Practice management |
| 7 | Academic | | |
| 8 | Staff | Collaborative task | Practice management |
| 9 | Primary health care | Case discussion | |
| 10 | Review | Supervision | Practice management |
| 11 | Academic | | |
| 12 | Staff | Collaborative task | Practice management |
| 13 | Primary health care | | |
| 14 | Process | Supervision | Practice management |
| 15 | Academic | Case discussion | |
| 16 | Staff | | Practice management |
| 17 | (Free) | Collaborative task | |
| 18 | Primary health care | | Practice management |
| 19 | Process | Supervision | |
| 20 | Academic | | Practice management |
| 21 | Staff | Collaborative task | |
| 22 | Primary health care | Case discussion | Practice management |
| 23 | Process | Supervision | |
| 24 | Academic | | Practice management |
| 25 | Staff | Collaborative task | |
| 26 | Primary health care | | Practice management |
| 27 | AGM | Supervision | |
| 28 | Academic | Case discussion | Practice management |
| 29 | Staff | | |
| 30 | (Free) | Collaborative task | Practice management |
| 31 | (Free) | | |
| 32 | (Free) | | |
| 33 | (Free) | | |
| 34 | (Free) | | |

**Figure 5.6**   Profile of counsellors' team and network meetings over one year (*cont'd*)

| Week (Jan–Dec) | Wednesday lunchtime meetings | Counsellors and counsellor/GP meetings | Other meetings with counsellor representation |
|---|---|---|---|
| 35 | Primary health care | | Practice management |
| 36 | Process | Supervision | |
| 37 | Academic | Case discussion | Practice management |
| 38 | Staff | | |
| 39 | (Free) | Collaborative task | Practice management |
| 40 | Primary health care | | |
| 41 | Process | Supervision | Practice management |
| 42 | Academic | Case discussion | |
| 43 | Staff | Collaborative task | Practice management |
| 44 | Primary health care | | |
| 45 | Review | Supervision | Practice management |
| 46 | Academic | | |
| 47 | Staff | Collaborative task | Practice management |
| 48 | Primary health care | Case discussion | |
| 49 | Process | Supervision | Practice management |
| 50 | Academic | | |
| 51 | Staff | Collaborative task | Practice management |
| 52 | (Free) | | |

*Key*
*Wednesday lunchtimes*
Primary health care team meeting (multi-professional and inter-agency network)
Process meeting (health centre clinical staff)
Academic meeting (multi-professional team and Centre for Community Care and Primary
    Health)
Staff meeting (clinical and administrative staff)
Review: four-monthly review meeting (multi-professional, inter-agency, university)
AGM: annual general meeting (multi-professional, inter-agency, university)

*Counsellors and counsellor/GP meetings*
Collaborative task meeting (counsellors and GPs)
Supervision (counsellor and supervisor)
Case discussion meeting (counselling team manager)

*Other meetings with counsellor representation*
Practice management meeting (GPs, practice manager, unit managers)

**Figure 5.7**  Profile of two counsellors' sessions over one year

**Counsellor 1**

| | 1 | 2 | 3 | 4 | 5 | 6 | 7 | 8 | 9 | 10 | 11 | 12 | 13 | 14 | 15 | 16 | 17 |
|---|---|---|---|---|---|---|---|---|---|---|---|---|---|---|---|---|---|
| 11.00 (50 mins) | D1 | S | D3 | M | M | S | D1 | M | D4 | S | D1 | M | D4 | H | H | D1 | M |
| 10.30 (30 mins) | | X1 | X1 | C3 | C1 | D5 | | E2 | E2 | E2 | E2 | E2 | E2 | H | H | H | D5 |
| 9.30 (50 mins) | C1 | C1 | C1 | C3 | C1 | C3 | C1 | C3 | C6 | C3 | C6 | C3 | C6 | H | H | C6 | |
| 8.30 (50 mins) | B1 | B1 | B1 | B1 | A2 | A2 | B4 | B4 | B4 | B4 | B4 | B4 | B4 | H | H | B4 | B4 |
| Week | 1 | 2 | 3 | 4 | 5 | 6 | 7 | 8 | 9 | 10 | 11 | 12 | 13 | 14 | 15 | 16 | 17 |
| Month | Jan | | | | Feb | | | | Mar | | | | Apr | | | | |

| | 18 | 19 | 20 | 21 | 22 | 23 | 24 | 25 | 26 | 27 | 28 | 29 | 30 | 31 | 32 | 33 | 34 |
|---|---|---|---|---|---|---|---|---|---|---|---|---|---|---|---|---|---|
| 11.00 (50 mins) | D1 | S | A6 | M | D4 | S | D1 | M | D4 | S | | D1 | M | D4 | H | H | D1 |
| 10.30 (30 mins) | D5 | D5 | FU | FU | D5 | | | FU | | D5 | D5 | | D5 | | H | H | D5 |
| 9.30 (50 mins) | C6 | B4 | C6 | A6 | C6 | A7 | A8 | B7 | B8 | B8 | B8 | B8 | B8 | B8 | H | H | B8 |
| 8.30 (50 mins) | B4 | B4 | B4 | B4 | FU | FU | B7 | B7 | B7 | B7 | B7 | B7 | B7 | B7 | H | H | B7 |
| Week | 18 | 19 | 20 | 21 | 22 | 23 | 24 | 25 | 26 | 27 | 28 | 29 | 30 | 31 | 32 | 33 | 34 |
| Month | May | | | | June | | | | July | | | | | Aug | | | |

| | 35 | 36 | 37 | 38 | 39 | 40 | 41 | 42 | 43 | 44 | 45 | 46 | 47 | 48 | 49 | 50 | 51 | 52 |
|---|---|---|---|---|---|---|---|---|---|---|---|---|---|---|---|---|---|---|
| 11.00 (50 mins) | D4 | S | A11 | D1 | M | D4 | S | D1 | M | FU | S | D4 | M | D1 | S | D4 | M | H |
| 10.30 (30 mins) | FU | D5 | D5 | | FU | | D5 | | | | D5 | | E5 | E5 | D5 | E5 | E5 | H |
| 9.30 (50 mins) | B8 | B8 | B8 | A11 | FU | C9 | C10 | C9 | C10 | C9 | C10 | C9 | C10 | C9 | C10 | A14 | A14 | H |
| 8.30 (50 mins) | B7 | B7 | B7 | B7 | FU | B11 | B11 | B11 | B11 | B11 | B11 | B11 | B11 | B11 | B11 | B11 | B11 | H |
| Week | 35 | 36 | 37 | 38 | 39 | 40 | 41 | 42 | 43 | 44 | 45 | 46 | 47 | 48 | 49 | 50 | 51 | 52 |
| Month | Sept | | | | | Oct | | | | Nov | | | | Dec | | | | |

## Counsellor 2

### Weeks 1–17 (Jan–Apr)

| Time | 1 | 2 | 3 | 4 | 5 | 6 | 7 | 8 | 9 | 10 | 11 | 12 | 13 | 14 | 15 | 16 | 17 |
|---|---|---|---|---|---|---|---|---|---|---|---|---|---|---|---|---|---|
| 16.30 (50 mins) | B3 | B3 | B3 | B3 | A1 | A3 | A3 | A3 | B5 | B5 | B5 | B5 | H | B5 | B5 | B5 | B5 |
| 15.30 (50 mins) | C2 | S | C2 | A1 | C2 | S | C2 | C2 | C2 | S | C2 | D3 | H | S | FU | D3 | A4 |
| 15.00 (30 mins) |  | D2 |  | E1 | E1 | E1 | E1 | E1 | E1 | E1 |  | D3 | H |  | FU |  | X2 |
| 14.00 (50 mins) | B2 | B2 | B2 | B2 | B2 | C4 | C5 | C4 | C5 | C4 | C5 | C4 | H | C5 | FU | C5 | A5 |
| Week | 1 | 2 | 3 | 4 | 5 | 6 | 7 | 8 | 9 | 10 | 11 | 12 | 13 | 14 | 15 | 16 | 17 |
| Month | Jan |  |  |  | Feb |  |  |  | Mar |  |  |  | Apr |  |  |  |  |

### Weeks 18–34 (May–Aug)

| Time | 18 | 19 | 20 | 21 | 22 | 23 | 24 | 25 | 26 | 27 | 28 | 29 | 30 | 31 | 32 | 33 | 34 |
|---|---|---|---|---|---|---|---|---|---|---|---|---|---|---|---|---|---|
| 16.30 (50 mins) | B6 | B6 | B6 | B6 | B6 | B6 | B6 | B6 | B6 | B6 | B6 | H | H | B9 | B9 | B9 | B9 |
| 15.30 (50 mins) | A4 | S | D3 | C7 | C7 | S | C7 | A9 | C7 | S | E3 | H | H | A10 | A10 | C7 | FU |
| 15.00 (30 mins) | X2 |  |  |  |  |  | E3 | E3 | E3 | E3 | E3 | H | H | E3 | E3 | E3 |  |
| 14.00 (50 mins) | C5 | FU | C5 | A7 | C5 | C8 | C5 | A8 | C8 | C8 | C8 | H | H | D6 | C8 | C8 | D6 |
| Week | 18 | 19 | 20 | 21 | 22 | 23 | 24 | 25 | 26 | 27 | 28 | 29 | 30 | 31 | 32 | 33 | 34 |
| Month | May |  |  |  | June |  |  |  | July |  |  |  |  | Aug |  |  |  |

### Weeks 35–52 (Sept–Dec)

| Time | 35 | 36 | 37 | 38 | 39 | 40 | 41 | 42 | 43 | 44 | 45 | 46 | 47 | 48 | 49 | 50 | 51 | 52 |
|---|---|---|---|---|---|---|---|---|---|---|---|---|---|---|---|---|---|---|
| 16.30 (50 mins) | B9 | B9 | B9 | B10 | B10 | B10 | B10 | B10 | B10 | B10 | A12 | A12 | A13 | A13 | B12 | B12 | B12 | H |
| 15.30 (50 mins) | D7 | S | D8 | FU | D7 | D8 | S | D7 | D8 | D9 | S | D8 | D10 | D9 | D9 | S | D8 | H |
| 15.00 (30 mins) | E3 |  |  |  | FU | E4 | E4 | E4 | E4 | E4 |  |  |  | FU | X3 | X3 | X3 | H |
| 14.00 (50 mins) | C8 | D6 | C8 | FU | C8 | D6 | C8 | C11 | C8 | C11 | D6 | C11 | C11 | C11 | D6 | C8 | C11 | H |
| Week | 35 | 36 | 37 | 38 | 39 | 40 | 41 | 42 | 43 | 44 | 45 | 46 | 47 | 48 | 49 | 50 | 51 | 52 |
| Month | Sept |  |  |  |  | Oct |  |  |  | Nov |  |  |  | Dec |  |  |  |  |

Key
A  1 or 2 50-minute sessions (N = 14)
B  Assessment plus 10 weekly 50-minute sessions (N = 12)
C  Assessment plus 10 fortnightly 50-minute sessions (N = 11)
D  Assessment plus 30-minute or 50-minute sessions from time to time (N = 10)
E  Assessment plus up to 10 30-minute weekly or fortnightly sessions (N = 5)
X  Emergency 30-minute sessions (N = 3)

Regular non-clinical events
M  Meetings
S  Supervision
H  Holiday

## Managing the workload

To illustrate the way the counsellors manage their time, Figure 5.7 shows two three-and-a-half-hour sessions of counselling time over a typical year. Each counsellor makes different use of the four counselling slots available to her, improvising and planning her time according to the pattern of routine meetings and the diverse needs of the counselling referrals that come her way. Using the menu of counselling services to plan their time allows these two counsellors to capitalize on their individual strengths and weaknesses, Counsellor 1 having greater strengths with complex, longer term cases, and Counsellor 2 with focused brief work.

Reading from bottom to top, the columns provide name of month, number of week, and four counselling slots, each one consisting of three fifty-minute slots and one thirty minute slot. The letters stand for Services A–E and Service X and the numbers by them stand for each patient. Thus column 1 for Counsellor 1 shows the first week in January, with one session each for the first patients of the year for Services B and C (B1 and C1), a half-hour administration slot, and the first patient of the year for Service D (D1).

- Counsellor 1. For this counsellor, the first slot of the morning is mostly given over to Service B (brief weekly work) and Service D (open-ended intermittent sessions), with Service A (one or two exploratory sessions) fitting in where possible. The next slot holds for the most part two Service C patients, changing to Service B as the need arises. The third slot is thirty minutes in length and is made up of approximately half clinical work (Service E, D or X/emergency) and half administration and liaison. The morning ends with a slot in which monthly meetings, monthly supervision and Service D rotate.
- Counsellor 2. For this counsellor, the first slot of the afternoon mostly holds two Service C patients, again changing to Service B as the need arises, and for a period rotating Service D patients around one Service C patient. The second hour is the thirty-minute slot, something under half of which is used for administration/liaison, the remaining time for Service E and the occasional emergency (Service X). The third hour also rotates, in this instance between supervision and Services D, C and A. The fourth hour accommodates the weekly Service B and occasionally Service A.

In the context of a setting which can often seem chaotic and rushed, the potential of the Menu of Services for a flexibility that is also structured and considered is of clear benefit. The discipline involved in managing case-loads is shared by GPs, who have to use time very economically in the ten-minute slots which are the standard patient appointments. This shared sense of the value of time can make for good working relations between the different professionals in the team.

The final section of this chapter looks briefly at developing the management of referrals for counselling.

## MANAGING COUNSELLING AS A GENERAL PRACTICE RESOURCE: A PROACTIVE RESPONSE TO DIVERSE NEEDS

The policy shift towards empowerment of patients and accountability as a key factor in the relationship between purchaser and provider has led to changes in the way in which referrals are made (see Chapter 3). Instead of reacting to what comes their way, the counsellors now provide information to GPs and patients that enables more informed choices to be made about how they use counsellors' time. The Menu of Counselling Services has provided a way to measure patient demand against a finite resource.

Developing the Menu will enable the counsellors to provide GPs with annual 'quotas', a form of internal contract that makes choices about patterns of work more transparent. GPs will then be able to make decisions about which of the many possible counselling referrals should be put through on the basis of need and appropriateness as well as of availability. If Dr A, for example, knows that she can refer five patients for weekly work (Service B) in a year, and in August has used up three of these, she will need to prioritize any further requests for that service with great care. A further development is for a named GP to take overall charge of counselling referrals, which will make it possible for members of the GP team to negotiate with each other over possible swaps and barters, a development that is likely to sharpen referral skills and knowledge and to enhance a sense of the practical aspects of the managerial relationship with the counselling team.

## IN CONCLUSION . . .

Counselling in general practice is, like playing jazz, a highly disciplined group activity. If done well, it can seem fluid and easy, instilling confidence in the patients and encouraging them to play an active part in the process of shaping the managerial routines of the GP and the counsellor.

The Menu of Counselling Services from which the patient is asked to choose can be thought of as one of the repeated elements in jazz, the harmonies and rhythms over which all the practitioners improvise, always listening and responding to the patients' voices and to the themes and motifs they introduce. This combination of structure and free play allows the team to respond to each individual's need for containment, rather than constantly reacting to pressure from outside, or imposing a rigidly held set of treatments from within.

In summary, this profile of the counselling year shows that:

- audit is of value as a research and management tool for counselling in general practice
    — features of internal audit designed for a particular setting provide opportunity for reflection on practice and on resource management
    — the Leeds CORE system data will provide a national picture of counselling process and outcome
- the problems brought to inner city general practices reflect wider social change, on local, national and global levels
- doctors' appointments accommodate the random presentations of patients within a highly structured time frame
- counsellors' own time frames and the paradox of planned but flexible provision can provide a structured response to fluctuating referral rates
- government policy increasingly demands transparent management and the most economic use of limited resources.

Balint (1964), while acknowledging the inevitability of an apostolic function in the GP which led him to want to 'convert ... all the ignorant and unbelieving among his patients', encouraged doctors to be 'elastic and adaptable enough to allow a great variety of relationships to develop between [the GP] and his patients' (p. 217). By identifying and developing the potential for both improvisation and routine, the counsellors, rather than expecting to convert the practice to their own existing ways of working, try, like Schön's 'reflective practitioner', to 'feel where the music is going and adjust their playing accordingly'. In this way, they play their own distinctive part in the complex ensemble work of the multi-professional team.

# Working debates ... the literature ... the theory ... the discussions

## Introduction

One must regard any theory as tentative, subject to error, and likely to be disconfirmed; one must be suspicious of it.

Chris Argyris and Donald Schön, *Theory in practice: increasing professional effectiveness*

Part 2 tackles the conceptual and evidence-base for our work. The title 'Working debates ... the literature ... the theory ... the discussions' was chosen because, as with the clinical material in Part 3, we wanted to give a sense of how such material is always living and imperfect and constantly under review; constantly 'rewritten' as the multi-professional team changes or grows. Our aim has been to highlight this sense of continuous reinterpretation because it gives some sense of the dynamic nature of debate in a very mixed team. That said, though influenced by the team in which we work, we are of course giving our own version of the literature, the theory and the discussions.

In Chapter 6 key issues in the expanding literature on counselling in the inner city in general practice and in primary care are addressed. At the time of writing, a new Labour government was in the midst of recasting the massive changes that had taken place under the conservative administration since 1990. Primary Care Groups (PCGs) have been established to develop local management of services for populations of about 100 000. Government bodies will ensure PCGs are working to evidence-based practice. The place of counselling is uncertain. On the one hand, one Health Minister has said he wants to see 'a counsellor in every practice'; on the other, counsellors do not have a place on the primary care group executives, although there is a GP responsible for mental health. In central London the PCG is complex, being built from collaboration between about twenty seven practices and their adjacent community health, social services and voluntary sector organizations. Any move towards geographical coterminosity between health and social services will help reduce the daunting complexity of the inter-agency network that can be involved in the care of any one individual with a variety of different needs.

Chapter 7, 'Reflective practice and the post modern context', is in some ways a core chapter. It summarizes our central conceptual framework for understanding the inner city context and the dilemmas facing not only counsellors, but any professional working in such complex conditions. It also provides a rationale for the pragmatic approach to counselling in general practice taken at Marylebone Health Centre, and for the 'local story' approach that we have taken in this book. The abstract ideas are presented here in pure form and then applied in future chapters. Most importantly, these ideas have motivated the attempt to establish a shared language in the multi-professional team, through the health centre's academic meetings, thus helping the team to move from a multi- to an inter-professional approach, with active collaboration across recognized professional differences. Our way of writing in Part 3, using direct rather than reported speech wherever possible, was also motivated by these ideas.

In Chapter 8, 'Theory in use: perspectives on containment', a conceptual building block which is much used in counselling and in other forms of therapeutic practice is examined, first abstractly and then through the 'grounded' or common language forged in the academic meetings. Here the business of reinterpreting and rewriting theory-in-practice is opened up, showing how difficult and complex it is for professionals to understand each other and to work together across their different languages, conceptual frameworks and belief systems. The second half of this chapter shows the multi-professional team trying to put the reflective practice philosophy to use, and acknowledging that they work in a postmodern context where superficial language games, including professional jargon, too easily render human distress banal and strip helplessness and despair of emotional meaning, often in order to protect the workers from their patients' sense of helplessness or confusion. We suggest that such social defences have to be opened up and re-examined in order to avoid the construction of a professional thick skin as well as to keep communication between professions on track (Menzies-Lyth 1988).

# 6

# Key themes in the literature on counselling in general practice

*Alison Vaspe*

The 'baby' of interprofessional work is at present separately represented by the different languages we use to describe our own individual work.

Patrick Pietroni, *Innovation in community care and primary health: the Marylebone experiment*

## SYNOPSIS

This chapter offers an overview of the working debates regarding counselling in general practice. It covers four key themes that recur in the literature:

- the extent and nature of counselling provision
- the role of counsellors in the general practice team
- the nature of the work
- audit, evaluation and research.

However, because counsellors in inner city general practices are usually accountable to doctors, whose changing conditions affect the counselling service itself, the chapter begins with a brief history of the key changes in primary care provision.

## THE PRIMARY CARE SETTING: A HISTORY OF CHANGE

There is a developing body of literature on counselling in general practice. From the 1970s, texts were appearing that described the experiences of individual counsellors and psychotherapists finding their way into what was an unfamiliar and challenging setting (e.g. Marsh & Barr 1975, Brook & Temperley 1976). In the 1990s a number of books by experienced general practice counsellors have appeared (Burton 1998, Wiener & Sher 1998, Corney & Jenkins 1993, East 1995, Keithley & Marsh 1995 and Lees 1999), yet as recently as 1996 counselling in general practice could be described as a 'relatively new innovation about which little is yet known' (Sibbald et al 1996a).

One reason for the difficulty of describing the work of counsellors in primary care as a generic activity lies in the wide variety of counselling practitioners involved (Sibbald et al 1993). Another is the problem of finding a language to convey the purpose and practice of counselling to non-counselling professionals (Pietroni P 1996b). However, counsellors are not alone in having to rethink, and to some extent standardize, their practice to meet the demands of the setting. All members of the primary care team have had to make significant and substantial changes to their roles and functions over the last decade or so. These changes have had their greatest impact on GPs themselves.

## Key developments in the primary care team

Since the founding of the NHS in 1948, several ideological and policy shifts in government have altered the way in which primary care is offered (Fig. 6.1). From an independent and often isolated role as individuals working from their own premises, often idiosyncratic in their specialities and treatments, general practitioners are now heading towards a phase of increasing orthodoxy and of accountability to what one commentator has described as 'an NHS inspectorate, seemingly modelled on Ofsted' (Klein 1998). This follows a period which has encouraged and emphasized patients' rights, including the right to sue those responsible for their care and the right to choose alternative treatments; there is also an increased emphasis on the individual's duty to take responsibility for, and control over, their own health (Pietroni P 1996a).

East (1995) has described how most of the first wave of GPs worked in isolation, even from health visitors and district nurses, and funded any developments in their practice from their own income. The concept of a primary care team was developed in the 1950s, to mixed reactions from the practitioners involved. Counsellors made a formal appearance on the scene in 1966, in the Family Doctors' Charter, which included them as members of ancillary staff whose salaries could be refunded by health authorities. However, most counsellors were either unpaid or were funded by a range of bodies and schemes including health promotion clinics, private health insurers and the National Marriage Guidance Council (now Relate).

Two other significant changes affecting the primary care team came about in the 1970s and 1980s. Further integration of nurses and health visitors into the primary care team was a feature of the reorganization of the NHS in 1974, which continued the trend of looking to preventive aspects of health care, while the rights of patients were brought into sharper focus by changes to the Mental Health Act in 1983. Davidson et al (1997) compare the growth of primary care counselling in the 1990s to the growth of community mental health teams in the 1980s, and also note the effect of the Care Programme Approach (CPA), implementation of which led to a decrease in the number of patients who could be treated by the community teams: 'it was [...] as a result of pressure from GPs following CPA that there has been the rapid growth of counselling to the point where there can be few parts of the country where the provision of counselling as a top-down initiative is not being actively considered' (p. 1). Direct reimbursement of counsellors was instituted in 1990, when GPs were allowed to claim a majority of counsellors' salaries from newly created Family Health Service Authorities (formerly Family Practitioner Committees). FHSAs were 'charged with improving the range, quality, cost effectiveness and consumer responsiveness of the family practitioner services component' (Huntington 1993, p. 303). As well as counselling, they also funded complementary therapy treatments and a range of preventive and early detection measures.

A major shift in attitude towards the NHS occurred during Margaret Thatcher's Conservative government, with the ending of the consensus view, held since Clement Attlee's post-war Labour government, of a welfare state that would provide health care for all, regardless of ability to pay. The NHS and Community Care Act (DoH 1990) placed the health service within a market framework. Hospital trusts and fundholding general practice surgeries provided a framework for costed episodes of care and a changed designation which recast patients as customers or consumers and their health and social care workers, including doctors, as purchasers and providers (Pietroni M 1995). With the new purchasing role of GPs as fundholders, doctors faced the challenge of an entirely new way of thinking about their work: gone was the professional autonomy they had traditionally enjoyed; in its place was the notion of a managed service with new accountabilities, particularly to financial management, audited quality measures, and inter-professional and inter-agency collaboration. A bewildering range of factors now had to be taken into account during any decision-making process, and negotiated in a plethora of professional languages (Pietroni P 1996b). Chapter 7 explores the different discourses surrounding patient care in the philosophical and historical context of postmodernism, and the implications for counsellors working in this setting.

A government initiative that was to have an impact on general practice in London was the Tomlinson Report. Set up in October 1991 to look into the capital's health services, medical education and research, the report proposed radical changes to the usage and provision of secondary health care. Recommendations included closure of some hospitals and mergers of others. Proposals for rationalization of hospital beds signalled a switch from secondary to primary care, although the King's Fund data on which these recommendations were made were seriously challenged by a leading London GP and epidemiologist, Brian Jarman (1983, 1984, 1988), the originator of the Underprivileged Area Score (UPAS). One direct effect for general practice was enhanced staffing as a result of money from London

---

**Figure 6.1**  Key policies affecting primary care in the 1990s

**Under the Conservative government of 1979–97**

1983 Mental Health Act
- community care
- closures of mental hospitals leading to bed shortages
- conflicts between patient rights and protection of community

1987 White Paper: *Promoting better health*
- promotion of good health
- emphasis on complete family health service

1989 *Working for patients*
- separation of health care funding from provision
- budgets held by GPs/health authorities

1990 NHS and Community Care Act
- market approach to care including NHS Trusts and GP fundholders
- non-medically qualified managers
- measurable outcomes

1991 White Paper: *The health of the nation*
- prevention and screening
- health targets in key areas
- demographic view
- inter-sector collaboration on public health education

1991 The Patient's Charter
- user-centred
- needs-based
- right to access to information
- public accountability

1992 Tomlinson Report
- loss of hospital beds in the capital city
- LIZEIs
- LATS
- funds for new focus on primary care

1996 White Paper: *Choice and opportunity*
- local flexibility
- independent practitioner contracts

1996 White Paper: *A service with ambition*
- working across team boundaries
- seamless service delivery
- prescribing integration
- nurses as gatekeepers
- performance reviews

1996 White Paper: *Delivering the future*
- nurse prescribers
- summative assessment
- research and development in primary care
- local and national IT networks

---

Implementation Zone Educational Initiatives (LIZEIs), with the appointment of young doctors as London Academic Training Scheme Fellows (LATS).

---

**Figure 6.1**   Key policies affecting primary care in the 1990s (*cont'd*)

**Under the Labour government elected in 1997**

1997 White Paper: *The new NHS: modern–dependable*
- Primary care groups (PCG)
  - — local authority collaboration
  - — community nursing
  - — multi-professional membership
- quality and performance initiatives

1998 Green Paper: *Our healthier nation*
- Health Improvement Plans (HIP)
- health authority and PCG collaboration
- local targets

1998 Health Action Zones announced through press releases and public information systems

1998 Action Paper: *Modernizing health and social services*
- reflecting needs of users, not institutions
- investment for reform
- modernization, management and local action
- reducing incidence of avoidable illness
- effective treatment on the basis of need alone
- maximize social development of children within stable family settings
- enable people with chronic illness, disability, or terminal illness to live lives as full and normal as possible

---

Benefits accrued to London general practices like Marylebone Health Centre, with its partnership with the University of Westminster, in terms of enhanced GP staffing and research. However, such short term posts also increased the sense of instability and complexity in the system. For counsellors, this meant a larger team of doctors, who on the whole they knew less well, referring from part-time posts. More broadly, the combined impact of the market framework and the closure of local hospitals and accident and emergency departments, along with rapid throughput of patients following surgery, resulted in vulnerable patients falling into what East describes as 'the gaps between said policies and done policies' (1995 p. 134).

However, the pace of change, already dramatic, was to accelerate again in May 1997 when a Labour landslide saw the election of Tony Blair as Prime Minister. He made a number of pledges to the nation based on a renewed commitment to social justice. In 1997 the white paper *The New NHS: modern–dependable* (DoH 1997) set out the Labour government's plans for primary and secondary care provision. In March 1999, fundholding and the internal market were abolished and existing general practices joined together in geographically based Primary Care Groups (PCGs), each catering for a patient population of approximately 100 000. These operate at one of four levels, which determine how much control they have over their budgets.

The plan is for PCGs eventually to commission all local health services, including mental health services. They will be in charge of budgets of up to £50 million (Curtis Jenkins 1998b). The ways they spend this money will be determined by local health improvement plans drawn up according to community based needs assessment. However, the approach to treatment will increasingly be expected to meet national standards of quality and performance, monitored by four bodies.

- A National Institute for Clinical Excellence (NICE) will take a lead on clinical and cost effectiveness.
- A clinical governance system will limit treatments on offer to those known and shown to be effective.
- A Commission for Health Improvement (CHI or CHIMP) will ensure that local systems maintain, assure and improve clinical standards.
- National service frameworks will provide frameworks for setting standards and defining service models in particular areas including mental health.

A dramatic change has taken place in the relationship between doctors and society. Gone is the old arrangement whereby the medical profession enjoyed autonomy, authority and self-regulation in return for providing a service for which the public had unquestioning respect and gratitude. The new exchange is based instead on national standards of quality performance in a climate of public accountability and proven effectiveness. The key policy aims are collaboration, cooperation, evidence-based treatment and health promotion at the local community level.

In the new NHS, GPs will be expected to adapt their practice to provide a more consistent form of primary health care to their patients, and counsellors, similarly, will be expected to justify their contribution.

## THE EXTENT AND NATURE OF COUNSELLING PROVISION

The advent of fundholding saw a dramatic increase in the numbers of counsellors directly employed by GPs. By 1996, 53% of the larger fundholding practices had counsellors in their surgeries, as opposed to 29% of non-fundholders (Corney 1996). A practical handbook published by the Leeds MIND Counselling in Primary Care Project (Rain 1997) found that for every 1000 patients in the city of Leeds there were between two and four-and-a-half hours of counselling in primary care available per week.

This increase has been justified on the grounds of statistics showing that, at any one point in time:

- the rate of mental illness in the overall population is between 10 and 15% (Mann 1993)

- up to 40% of those consulting their GP have a probable psychiatric disorder (Dowrick 1992)
- around 30% of the overall population will at some point have experienced symptoms of anxiety or depression (Dowrick 1992)
- in 1971 the cost of working days lost through mental illness, including statutory sick pay and invalidity benefits, was 0.4% of GDP; in 1991 these costs had increased to 1.3% of GDP, or £7314 million (Rain 1997)
- a referral to a psychiatric outpatients department costs upwards of three times the cost of referral to a counsellor in general practice, while clinical outcomes are equivalent and patient satisfaction is increased in the latter (Webber, Davies & Pietroni 1996).

As Mann (1993) observes, the primary care service is the main point of contact, not just for non-psychotic disorders (anxiety and depression), but often for people with psychiatric disorders.

None the less, the increase in counselling activity, despite the general satisfaction expressed by GPs, has given rise to debate and some concern. One area that has caused concern is the adequacy of the training of the various professionals involved. An early review of the field (Wylde 1981) showed that counselling might be provided by one or more of five professional groups: social workers, clinical psychologists, psychotherapists, marriage guidance counsellors and other counsellors. More recently, in a breakdown of the personnel involved in one thousand five hundred and forty two practices in England and Wales, Sibbald et al (1993) revealed that four hundred and eighty four (31%) had one or more people undertaking counselling as a distinct activity. Of these, one hundred and eighty one were community psychiatric nurses, one hundred and thirty four were generic counsellors and ninety five were clinical psychologists. The remaining seventy four practices had a variety of staff undertaking counselling, including GPs, practice nurses and health visitors.

Most counsellors in these studies were paid for directly by their practices or by the family health services or district health authority. Some were self-employed and paid by the patients themselves, while others were provided by independent counselling agencies with service contracts for several different practices in an area.

In 1984 the 'hotchpotch' of personnel offering their services was identified as the key problem of counselling in general practice (Rowland & Irving 1984). Over a decade later, Corney (1997) noted that the range of training and years and nature of experience of practice remained mixed and variable, while Roth and Fonagy (1996) found that counselling as a term was 'poorly defined both in clinical practice and in the research literature' (p. 255).

In 1988 a report for the Royal College of General Practitioners evaluating the work of counsellors in general practice found training could include marital and psychosexual specialities, psychotherapy, social work and family therapy, behavioural therapy and psychiatric nursing, as well as one- or two-year counselling courses at polytechnic or university (McLeod 1988). In 1994 a report on counselling in the Kensington, Chelsea and Westminster area revealed an array of diplomas, postgraduate degrees and substantial psychotherapy qualifications among practice counsellors, with 95% receiving regular supervision (Hicks 1994). This local study found that 95% of counsellors in the area had counselling qualifications, and 55% were accredited by the British Association for Counselling (BAC). This compares with the finding of a survey of primary care counsellors' experiences of supervision (Burton et al 1998) that, of the 71% sample of generic counsellors (as opposed to counselling psychologists, social workers, psychotherapists and nurses or CPNs), only 12% were BAC accredited. However, counselling training has been an area of rapid growth, and preliminary results from a contemporary national survey (Mellor-Clark 1998), involving nearly one thousand counsellors working in primary care, show that 90% hold both a certificate and a diploma in counselling.

## PROFESSIONAL ORGANIZATIONS AND SPECIAL INTEREST GROUPS

Counsellors in primary care are represented by several effective professional organizations. Two in particular have acted as a centre of gravity: the Counselling in Medical Settings (CMS or BACCMS) division of the BAC and the Counselling in Primary Care Trust (CPCT).

The BAC has responded to concerns regarding standards and safeguards in counselling on two levels: by adapting their accreditation procedures and by setting up a voluntary register of accredited counsellors (United Kingdom Register of Counsellors), membership of which will, for example,

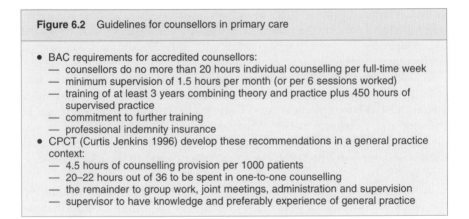

**Figure 6.2** Guidelines for counsellors in primary care

- BAC requirements for accredited counsellors:
  — counsellors do no more than 20 hours individual counselling per full-time week
  — minimum supervision of 1.5 hours per month (or per 6 sessions worked)
  — training of at least 3 years combining theory and practice plus 450 hours of supervised practice
  — commitment to further training
  — professional indemnity insurance
- CPCT (Curtis Jenkins 1996) develop these recommendations in a general practice context:
  — 4.5 hours of counselling provision per 1000 patients
  — 20–22 hours out of 36 to be spent in one-to-one counselling
  — the remainder to group work, joint meetings, administration and supervision
  — supervisor to have knowledge and preferably experience of general practice

be a requirement for counsellors wanting to practise in other European Community countries. The BAC has also issued detailed guidelines for good practice (Fig. 6.2) including a recommendation that primary care counsellors should have completed a substantial training of three years and at least four hundred and fifty supervised hours and that they should be committed to further training (Ball 1993). The need for training to cover both theoretical understanding and practical skills is emphasized. As well as an excellent newsletter (*Counselling in practice*) and other publications, a consultation service and a research database (Counsel.Lit.) and website (http://www.cpct.co.uk), the CPCT has developed the BAC guidelines and has produced a curriculum for a postgraduate diploma in primary care counselling (Fig. 6.3), which can be used as a stepping stone leading to an MSc in primary and secondary care health settings.

---

**Figure 6.3** Curriculum for postgraduate training in primary care (Rain 1997 after Henderson 1993)

- Knowledge relating to working in primary care
  - anti-oppressive practice and multicultural issues
  - organizational/systemic and cultural context of primary care
  - ethical issues arising from primary care work
  - caseload management
  - audit and research skills for evaluating counselling process, impact and outcomes
  - research methodology for qualitative and new paradigm research studies
  - medical model of health
- Clinical knowledge
  - time-limited and focused counselling
  - post-traumatic stress
  - loss and grief
  - psycho-sexual counselling
  - medical conditions and treatment in relation to counselling
  - pharmacology in relation to counselling
  - violence
  - sexual abuse
  - families and couples
  - groupwork
- Interpersonal skills
  - teamwork
  - negotiating
  - assertiveness

---

Emphasizing both the particular areas of knowledge required of primary care counsellors, and the interpersonal skills they need to find their place in the multi-professional team, the CPCT curriculum goes some way to addressing what Roberts (1997) has identified as an oversight in professional training: 'It is sometimes assumed that any accredited counsellor or therapist is suitable to work in a medical setting without further training, or any consideration of how the therapeutic effectiveness may be conceived of by the patient, or by the other health professionals who may be involved.' She believes such training to be 'a minimum requirement for those working with people who may be seriously ill, or may continuously present their difficulties in a manner which the GP's interest or consultation time cannot accommodate' (p 86).

Together, CMS and CPCT also run annual conferences on counselling in primary care which encourage team participation by GPs, managers and other members of the practice team, as well as counsellors.

In 1993 the National Council for Vocational Qualifications set up an advice, guidance and counselling lead body to establish the competencies required in these areas. The CMS and CPCT have cooperated with this attempt to clarify the skills and competencies required of primary care counsellors and, from 1994, psychotherapists. However, Curtis Jenkins (1998a) of the CPCT has urged caution. He questions whether NVQs can describe and test for competence in such a way as to satisfy patients of a counsellor's worth or safety. Noting the tendency of self-regulating organizations to act as 'old-fashioned guilds', he proposed a professional organization of all those working as counsellors in primary care which would break down barriers preventing inter-professional education and information sharing. Accordingly, in October 1998 the CPCT launched The Association of Professional Counsellors and Psychotherapists in Primary Care (CPC) with the object of:

- acting as a professional body for counsellors and psychotherapists working in primary health care, including setting standards of excellence, providing ethical guidance and promoting good practice
- promoting the role of counsellors in primary health care training
- promoting good practice in counselling in primary health care and researching new ways of working for the benefit of the public.

## THE ROLE OF COUNSELLORS IN THE GENERAL PRACTICE TEAM

Guidelines on counselling in general practice follow the BAC in making a clear distinction between counsellors and the use of counselling skills by other members of the multi-professional team (Ball 1993, Hurd & Rowland 1991, Irving & Heath 1989).

### Counselling skills in GPs: the influence of Michael Balint

The Hungarian psychoanalyst Michael Balint made a seminal contribution to developing the potential of the doctor/patient relationship. His Utopian vision was of a world in which the specialists will know 'the advantages of relinquishing the role of superior, omniscient mentors, and [accept] the much more realistic and rewarding role of expert assistants to the general practitioner, who now remains in full charge of his patients' (1964 p. 286). Emphasizing the effect on the patient's emotional difficulties of 'the doctor as drug', he noted the importance of the GP's 'apostolic function' in identifying underlying emotional issues and allowing space and time for these to be heard. Accurate and timely diagnosis could prevent these issues from becoming 'organized' as chronic physical presentations. Working closely with his wife, Enid, he formulated the 'flash' (Balint E 1973), a moment of communication which made available for discussion the often disorganized presentations of patients to their GPs. The 'flash' technique is discussed in Chapter 8.

While acknowledging Balint's 'seminal work on doctor-patient interactions', Rowland, Irving and Maynard (1989) debated whether GPs should in fact take on the role of counsellor to their patients. They found a conflict of role; in contrast to the 'authoritative helper who defines and resolves the problem, directs the course of treatment and gives advice and support', the counsellor aims to enable 'the client to help himself'. The authors also identified a difficulty for doctors with 'practitioner flair': GPs perhaps did and said the right thing at the right time, but were then left without the resources or the skills to respond to the resulting 'flood of confidences reflecting underlying psychosocial problems'.

Enid Balint et al (1993) counter this argument. They observe that counselling emerged in a space created by two traditions: the Balint group, and the movement for attaching social workers to general practice. They highlight the role of the Balint group in GPs' decisions about whether to develop their relationship with patients suffering emotional problems, or whether to 'recognize and refer' (Harris 1987). They regret the implication that 'Balint belongs to history' and also the view that his method of studying general practice lacks relevance for contemporary GPs, describing the continuing value of Balint groups in helping GPs rethink aspects of their training in 'one-person' medicine with a view to developing their abilities to take on the demands of 'two-person' medicine, and the human relations involved in GP/patient consultations.

Finally, Launer (1994) formulated three levels of counselling that he identified as taking place in the general practice surgery where he worked. One was formal counselling, undertaken by professionals; the other two occurred in or as a consequence of routine GP consultations. He considered it important to acknowledge the amount of psychological help given by GPs, often drawing upon counselling or other therapeutic techniques, but perceived by the patient as good, attentive listening.

## Counsellors as part of the general practice team

McLeod (1988) identified both advantages and disadvantages for bringing counselling to general practice. She considered that the advantages out-weighed the disadvantages, and noted the following benefits to patients, practices and counsellors.

- The patient sees someone trusted and known in a familiar setting.
- There is reduced stigma, compared to psychiatric referral.
- The practice can see a reduction in prescribing rates.
- The GPs develop an understanding of patients' underlying needs.
- Counsellors have improved access to medical information.
- Counsellors see patients before difficulties become entrenched.
- There is more interchange between counsellors and members of the general practice team.

She also noted some disadvantages.

- Patients lose out on privacy and confidentiality may be breached.
- The practice will have practical difficulties such as lack of space.
- Counsellors are unfamiliar with the general practice setting.
- Counsellors can become 'infected' with the medical model and sacrifice 'the precious commodity of time for a rapid turnover of patients'.

### Communication in the team

The question of privacy and confidentiality has been much debated in the literature, together with its implications for the role of the counsellor in the general practice team. Dammers and Wiener (1995) put forward two dis-tinct models. The first centres on a 'secure frame' approach, emphasizing the separateness and primacy of the counsellor/client relationship; the sec-ond adopts a team approach in which the boundary of confidentiality is held by the practice team.

**The 'secure frame' approach.** This model centres on patients' right to pri-vacy and autonomy, and on maintaining a clear distinction between the counselling ethos, which prioritizes self-determination, and a medical oath based on the fundamental duty to save lives. Information about the coun-selling may be shared with the GP concerned following discussion with the client and ways may be found of working more holistically by discussing with GPs some of the issues raised in counselling, but counsellors 'adhere to their own model of confidentiality which does not allow for the disclo-sure of any identifiable information about a client to anyone other than the named GP, or other specified member of the clinical team who shares the care of the client' (Graham 1995; p. 252).

**The team approach.** By setting the confidentiality boundary around the team as a whole, rather than around the counselling relationship, the sec-ond model prioritizes the patient's relationship with the primary care team, with discussion taking place before, during and sometimes after counselling. By keeping in mind the relationships of both counsellor and patient with the organization as a whole, potential splits and divisions can be averted.

In 1996 Sibbald et al (1996a) carried out in-depth telephone interviews with a wide representative sample of English and Welsh general practitioners on the subject of their experience of working with counsellors. They found that GPs thought counsellors too often unwilling to share information about the goals, progress or outcomes of their work. This was, they noted, a direct result of protecting confidentiality within the counselling relationship rather than within the bounds of the team. They concluded that 'This model of working is alien to and possibly unworkable in general practice' (p. 16).

The preliminary results of the UK survey of counsellors working in primary care show that 27% of counsellors rarely if ever meet GPs or discuss patients with them. Curtis Jenkins (1998b) suggests that one reason for this could be the restricted hours worked by counsellors in general practice. He also notes that in some practices, even GPs have difficulty in meeting each other to discuss their work.

On a clinical level, Sher (1992) considers that 'dynamic teamwork' between the doctor and counsellor or psychotherapist can enable them to serve as 'a container of anxiety' for the patient. Jones et al (1994) also stress the importance of the inter-professional relationship. They explore the potential for understanding inherent in the 'Oedipal triangle' of the patient's relationship to a 'parental couple' of GP and counsellor and the ways in which the 'difficulties' of the team setting can also provide an opportunity to learn more about the patient.

The broader social and organizational implications of counsellors working in the particular context of general practice are beginning to be explored in more depth. Mackenzie (1996) draws upon the work of Isabel Menzies Lyth to look at the concept of boundaries and the nature of the different social defences in one GP surgery. Lees (1997) explores the ways in which the 'core interaction between client and therapist … is influenced by, and has an influence on, (a) the practice as a whole, (b) the staff in the practice, (c) other patients, families and the community at large, and (d) the supervisory relationship' (p. 35).

In the wider context of mental health care provision, the need for integration and multi-disciplinary working has been noted. Corney (1999) and Roth and Fonagy (1996) underline the importance of liaison between primary and secondary care professionals in order to prevent fragmentation of mental health services and also to aid appropriate referral to psychotherapy services when necessary, particularly given the finding that a small percentage of patients can be harmed by counselling. They consider it to be essential that counsellors are able to identify who is and who is not likely to benefit from counselling.

# THE NATURE OF THE WORK

## The range of problems referred for counselling

A key issue for counsellors working in the generalist setting of primary health care is the broad range of referrals they receive. Lees (1999) notes that, unlike other settings in which counselling is offered, patients are seen in the context of their whole life, rather than in relation to a primary task such as learning (schools, colleges etc.) or performance at work (staff counselling).

The range of presentations seen by a general practice counsellor extends from patients with serious physical illness to those suffering from long term mental health problems (Pietroni M 1999). In an overview of a sample of studies undertaken between 1975 and 1992, East (1995) found symptoms and conditions on presentation included:

- addiction
- psychosomatic disorders
- emotional distress
- anxiety
- depression
- neurotic disorders
- psychiatric illness.

External events included:

- interpersonal problems
- marital/relationship problems
- abortion
- stress linked to crisis and trauma
- sudden traumatic event
- reaction to receiving disturbing information in an abrupt manner in hospitals.

Among the GPs interviewed by Sibbald et al (1996a), the most common reasons for referring patients for counselling were:

- stress/anxiety (63% of practitioners)
- relationship problems (42%)
- depression (40%)
- bereavement (26%)
- phobias/obsessions (26%).

The level of severity is generally located somewhere between the occasional visitor to the surgery for specific and separate treatments, and a group of the more seriously mentally ill needing regular and ongoing support from community mental health teams. For example, in a study of sixty new counselling clients seen in a year, Marsh (1993) found that, compared with sixty patients of equivalent age and gender, the counselling clients both utilized medical services more frequently and represented a 'psychiatrically sicker group'. In 1996 the fifth St George's Conference on Counselling in Primary Care heard a report on a successful pilot project introducing counsellors into general practices (Sedgwick-Taylor 1996). The aim was for patients to receive in-house counselling for 'serious or relatively serious neurotic complaints, often arising from a life trauma and/or psychosocial problems ... though not mentally ill'. Community mental health team services could then be preserved for patients in the community whose psychotic or chronic depressive and/or anxiety conditions meant they needed ongoing care in order to continue to function.

Mann (1993) reviewed the research showing the extent of psychiatric and psychosocial disorder seen in primary care. He found the difficulties of patients with non-psychotic psychiatric disorders were often dismissed on the basis of such arguments as:

- not a major health issue in comparison with many common physical diseases
- not 'real' mental illnesses
- nothing much is known and anyway most of these disorders recover spontaneously.

He notes the significance in depression of a 'complex of social adversity' made up of limited and difficult relationships, personal vulnerability and adverse events. This emphasis on the role of 'important and meaningful life problems' is generally considered to be a factor in good outcomes (see Corney 1993, Wiener & Sher 1998). The potential effect on mental health of external events, alongside social isolation and individual susceptibility, is supported by a recent review (NHS Centre for Reviews and Dissemination 1997) which identified groups at high risk of long term mental health problems. For children, characteristics included:

- living in poverty
- experiencing parental separation and divorce
- in families experiencing bereavement.

For adults, they included:

- undergoing divorce or separation
- unemployed
- at risk of depression in pregnancy
- experiencing bereavement
- long term carers of people who are highly dependent.

The authors regretted the lack of research demonstrating counselling's effectiveness, especially when offered as a sole intervention, but noted the contribution of high quality, timely psychological intervention offered in conjunction with medical interventions such as anti-depressant medication. They encouraged health authorities to shape their commissioning of services accordingly.

## Factors in appropriate referral for brief, target counselling

Burton (1998) has provided a useful overview of the different models of counselling and psychotherapy in primary care (Box 6.4). She makes a thorough exploration of the factors involved in assessing for brief or longer term counselling and psychotherapy and notes the 'pressing question in the present cost-containment climate in health care': 'How much counselling or psychotherapy is enough for this patient?' (p. 53). The following discussion is based on the literature about brief, targeted counselling. Little has been written on longer-term, supportive work in primary care.

---

**Figure 6.4**   Models of counselling and psychotherapy in primary care (from Burton 1998, pp. 63–89)

- Mainstream
  — psychodynamic
  — cognitive behavioural (CBT)
  — humanistic
- Integrative
  — cognitive analytic therapy (CAT)
- Group, couple and family therapies (including psycho-sexual counselling)
- Single session and 2 + 1
- Other brief models
  — solution-focused
  — psychotherapy abbreviation
  — inter-personal-developmental-existential
  — brief intermittent psychotherapy throughout the life cycle

---

Burton et al (1998) found that most primary care counsellors in their sample offered brief, targeted counselling, although one third of their respondents said the number of sessions they could offer patients was unlimited. The average maximum was thirteen sessions. The Leeds handbook (Rain 1997), which was based on local, national and international data, also found that the most common form of counselling available in GP surgeries was brief and targeted. They summarized the conditions most amenable to this kind of counselling:

- life crisis (loss, trauma, sudden change)
- relationship difficulties
- anxiety and stress
- breakdown in coping

- depressive symptoms
- somatization
- high utilizers of medical services ('heartsink' patients)
- difficulties with pain management in conjunction with other medical treatment.

The UK Survey of counsellors in primary care found unplanned endings to occur in as many as 50% of cases. The Leeds CORE System (CORE System Group 1998) includes an option to evaluate outcome at the end of each session, rather than simply at the beginning and end of the counselling, while Booth et al (1997), in a study of fifteen practices in Shropshire's Mental Health NHS Trust, found that a surprising number of patients who did not complete their agreed period of work were none the less satisfied with the service they had received, some even reporting 'remarkable' life changes as a result.

David Malan, himself a student and colleague of Michael Balint, was among the first psychoanalytic practitioners to respond to limited resources, increasing demand and ever lengthening waiting lists by developing a time-limited model (Malan 1963, 1976a, 1976b, 1979). His brief therapy of thirty sessions is much more than most primary care counsellors offer but the principles behind his 'triangle of insight' (1979), and the factors that make this an appropriate treatment for patients (psychological mindedness, motivation, a focus for the work etc.), provide helpful and useable guidelines for those working in this setting, whether referring or counselling. Other key contributors to the literature are Mann (1973), Molnos (1995), Gustafson (1986, 1995a, 1995b), Feltham (1997) and Elton Wilson (1996), while the time-limited therapies developed by Mohamed and Smith (1997) at the Women's Therapy Centre in London include a transcultural model.

As well as drawing upon the psychoanalytic tradition, Mohamed and Smith note the effectiveness of cognitive analytic therapy (Ryle 1990) for patients contraindicated for brief psychodynamic work. Roth and Fonagy (1996) found the research literature showed cognitive behavioural therapy (CBT) to be an efficacious form of brief work (sometimes in conjunction with structured psychodynamic therapy) for certain conditions including anxiety disorders, depression and some phobias.

Contraindications for counselling have been identified on the basis of experience, although there is variation in practice and some counsellors may do better with particular presentations than others. However, there is substantial agreement that brief counselling is not generally appropriate for:

- serious emotional disturbance
- psychosis or dependency issues
- compulsive behaviour
- severe and entrenched depression

- patients seriously at risk of suicide
- longstanding eating disorders such as bulimia and anorexia.

(Dammers & Wiener 1995 p. 37)

Burton (1998 p. 61) identifies at least four potential negative outcomes of 'six sessions for everything':

- serious suicide attempt, when termination is perceived as abandonment
- patients are passed from one clinician to another for brief therapy while underlying issues are left unaddressed
- the patient may feel 'a little better but counselling didn't change anything' and may relapse or develop new symptoms
- the patient's deep-seated problems are managed by a clinician who has not had sufficient training and specialist intervention is needed.

Wiener and Sher (1998) make the point that brief work, though usually taken to mean six to twelve sessions, can be used more flexibly, with the frequency of sessions adapted to the needs of the patient. Andrew Elder, in his preface to their book, regrets the 'present unfortunate dominance' of six-session models which he considers to run against the open door nature of general practice and to be driven by anxieties about patients' unlimited need. He identifies a number of possibilities for counselling in general practice and concludes: 'the clinical parameters of work in this setting are still to be defined.'

## AUDIT, EVALUATION AND RESEARCH

Curtis Jenkins (1998a) has alerted counsellors in primary care to the chasms being opened up between health professionals and society. He identifies two problem areas that counsellors need to confront if they are to maintain the good relationship they have so far enjoyed with patients:

- the age-old problem of the NHS, of inadequate resources and rising public demand
- the problem of how to respond to the public demand for accountability and openness in the self-regulation of the profession.

Both the limited amount of funding available and the demand for accountability and openness put pressure on counsellors to show that they are offering a service that is value for money. Figure 6.5 lists the main forms of audit, evaluation and research methods being used by counsellors in general practice, ranging from the routine collection of data to the more sophisticated forms of treatment comparison in terms of efficacy and cost. Tolley and Rowland (1995) suggest that these different activities should go on alongside each other according to need: supervision and case discussion alongside the gathering of audit data, the micro-level of process research alongside the macro-level of outcome studies justifying requests for funding from employers and funding agencies.

---

**Figure 6.5**   Audit, research and evaluation of counselling in general practice (after Bond 1995, Tolley & Rowland 1995, Wiener & Sher 1998, Burton 1998).

- routine quantitative auditing
  - demographics
  - attendance
  - referral sources
  - presenting problems
- additional monitoring of qualitative factors, e.g.
  - service delivery (information provided before, during and after counselling, accessibility of the service etc.)
  - client participation (feedback and complaints)
  - staffing (training and experience, supervision arrangements, continuity of service)
  - cooperation and liaison with other members of the practice
- qualitative research, e.g.
  - case discussion
  - case histories
  - examination of specific issues (e.g. chronic illness, redundancy)
  - observational studies
  - process research
  - semi- or unstructured in-depth interviews
- evaluation outcome studies (measuring rate of change over a period of time), e.g.
  - clinical outcome (drop in symptom level, improved quality of life)
  - change in medical utilization rates (reduction in GP consultations, better use of consultations, reduction in prescribed medicines, reduced referrals to psychiatric and other services, reduced costs in managing patients)
  - patient satisfaction
  - randomized control trials (RCTs) measuring efficacy (rate of change against other treatments and a control group)
  - effectiveness studies ('naturalistic' studies based on data gathered in situ)
- economic evaluation (cost-minimization, cost-benefit, cost-effectiveness, cost utility analysis)

---

## Research questions and methodologies: the qualitative/quantitative debate

Most counsellors now accept the need to monitor the service they offer in terms of numbers of patients, sessions per patient and completed patient contracts (Corney 1999). There is also increasing interest among counsellors in carrying out research studies on counselling in primary care: the recently founded BAC research network (BAC 1998) has published a list of two hundred and eighty nine members, of whom over 10% (thirty four) specify this area as a research interest. However, the Leeds CORE team (CORE System Group 1998) have noted a gap between researchers and practitioners which they consider needs to be bridged before research can achieve its full potential as a tool for counsellors in general practice. They trace a series of overlapping research generations working to different agendas since the 1950s:

- 1950s–1970s: establishing the efficacy[1] of psychotherapy using control groups of patients receiving no formal intervention
- 1960s–1980s: trying to determine the most efficacious of the various brands of psychotherapy using randomized control trials (RCTs)
- 1970s–1990s: tackling the interface between efficacy research and real world service delivery and investigating issues of cost-effectiveness, therapy, 'dosage' (how much is needed) and allocation of resources to those most in need
- 1984 to present: a renewed focus on more exploratory approaches including process research and on attempts to see the patient in context. (CORE System Group 1998 pp. 17–18)

Broadly speaking, the debate is divided between traditional scientific methods which attempt to identify 'what works for whom' in 'the most ideal set of circumstances, delivered by the most ideal practitioners, to the most ideal patients, with the most ideal specificity and severity of problem' (Mellor-Clark, in Burton 1998. p. 164) and systematic but naturalistic field studies such as process research which shows 'what happens in the counselling process itself' (Wiener & Sher 1998 p. 146). Burton reviews the arguments very well, and sets the debate in the broader context outlined at the start of this chapter, in which the NHS as a whole will operate to best national standards of quality and performance.

The randomized control trial has its critics, not just among practitioners (e.g. Balint et al 1993, House 1997, Wiener & Sher 1998), but also among some general practitioners and medical researchers (Maynard 1995, Aldridge & Pietroni 1996). As Hughes (1996) notes, writing about the current trend towards evidence-based medicine, the response of the GP in the field when presented with empirical research, from which all atypical features have been carefully removed, is to point to the number of atypical patients he or she deals with day after day, protesting that 'a lot of individuals just do not fit your limiting criteria, and I still have to offer them treatment'. There is a need for art to sit alongside science, claims Hughes: 'Our understanding of illness and treatment is informed and illuminated by biology, but assessment is always undertaken in the light of the way an individual case presents, and needs not just an assessment of the scientifically verifiable facts, but of the presenting story, the patient's account of what has happened to bring her to consult the doctor' (p. 16).

---

[1] A distinction is made in the literature between *efficacy*, established through strictly controlled settings in conditions resembling laboratory trials, and *effectiveness*, found through gathering data on 'real' patients viewed in context.

The difficulty in finding a form of research that will do justice to counselling in primary care is compounded by a highly charged social dynamic of professional rivalry (Corney 1999). A combination of the different orientations of the various practitioners offering counselling and / or counselling skills in this setting, and the different languages and associated professional ways of thinking of others involved in the world of mental health care, compounds the difficulty in sustaining a regard for cumulative evidence that increases the 'core knowledge' of counselling in general practice, rather than aiming to 'prove a point' (Pietroni 1996c). Furthermore, the time-limited contracts of many of the personnel involved can reduce opportunities for a dialogue with purchasers that takes place over time (Sibbald et al 1996b) and for long term research studies to be carried through.

## Arguments for and against counselling in primary care

Reviewing published and unpublished research studies, Graham Curtis Jenkins (1995b) found that trained counsellors with sufficient experience, appropriate supervision and an integrated approach to the primary care team could achieve the following outcomes:

- 80–90% of patients seen between four and six times estimated counselling had been helpful or very helpful
- 20–50% of patients taking psychotropic drugs before counselling (around 33% of referrals) reported discontinuing or reducing medication after counselling
- consultation rates with GPs fell and remained lower for as long as six months following counselling.

In contrast:

- only 2–6% of patients found the experience unhelpful or very unhelpful
- only 2–6% of patients increased the dose of prescribed drugs following counselling.

In their 1996 study, Sibbald et al reviewed the evidence base underpinning reported advantages of providing counselling as a part of primary health care services. They found that research supported the contention that a majority of patients prefer in-house mental health professionals. However, they suggested that the areas identified by Curtis Jenkins need to receive systematic enquiry in terms of their impact on health outcomes and claimed that:

- descriptive evidence of reduced workload for GPs, reduced prescribing of psychotropic drugs and lower off-site referral rates was conflicting
- evidence from controlled trials did not support claims of reduced consultation rates or reductions in prescribing psychotropic drugs.

Roth and Fonagy (1996) included a chapter on counselling and primary care interventions in their review of the literature on the efficacy of different therapeutic treatments for defined patient populations. They noted the difficulty in assessing the efficacy of counselling as revealed through research studies because of 'the lack of specificity and control in studies, the diversity of the patient groups studied, the variation in treatments administered, and the heterogeneity of contrast treatments' (p. 261). However, Davidson et al (1998), while concurring with this, regret what they consider a premature judgement by many service providers – based on Roth and Fonagy and therefore on evidence that is acknowledged to be patchy – that counselling cannot demonstrate consistent benefit to patients. They describe current attempts to use randomized control trials to answer the question 'Does counselling work in primary care?' and note the difficulties in methodology that have been encountered, together with the limitations of RCTs when considering external validity. They then describe the work of the Psychological Therapies Research Centre at Leeds University in designing and piloting a standardized audit assessment evaluation and outcome tool (CORE System Group 1998). They suggest there is a need for a much broader baseline than pure clinical effectiveness, and for qualitative measures to be used alongside measurement of medical offset costs and outcome data.

## The current debate

Burton (1998) and Curtis Jenkins (1995b), among others, have suggested it is time to leave behind old-fashioned 'Does it work?' research in favour of new questions, asking 'Why, how, when and where does counselling work in primary care?' In similar vein, Corney (1999) identifies four research questions that 'urgently need to be investigated'.

- Who benefits most from counselling?
- Who might be harmed by counselling?
- Which therapies benefit which patients?
- What level of skill is needed in the counsellor for benefit to occur?

Corney acknowledges the considerable methodological difficulties in carrying out clinical trials in the general practice setting, as well as the increasing acceptability of qualitative techniques. None the less, she believes clinical trials are crucial, given that a high proportion of patients suffering from anxiety and depression recover without outside intervention. For counselling to demonstrate that it is a cost-effective treatment, she believes it needs to show a higher rate of improvement than would occur in spontaneous remission.

In the context of a government-led drive towards reliable, evidence-based medical treatment, and of high public demand and tight public sector budgeting, the need for research demonstrating the cost-effectiveness and efficiency of primary care counselling has been described as urgent. The parallel drive towards transparency of service provision and professional accountability also highlights the need for clear definition and rigorous regulation among the different professions offering counselling in this setting. However, the tensions between advocates of different forms of research on the effectiveness and efficacy of counselling obscure the need that also exists for good quality descriptions of the problems counsellors respond to in the context of a complex environment.

## IN CONCLUSION ...

The literature on counselling in general practice is patchy and uneven. Contributions from counsellors in the field are limited, largely because of the fragile, part-time nature of their employment. The different professional languages involved (of the various counselling trainings; of those coming from backgrounds such as nursing, social work or psychology who also offer counselling; of medical and other forms of research into the effects of counselling) have made it difficult for the voices of those involved to do more than provide a series of often useful, but also often conflicting, individual accounts.

Up until now, GPs have taken the lead in assessing and evaluating the services being offered, with the result that a bio-medical language dominates the debate, while literature on the containment offered by the multiprofessional team and inter-agency network is virtually non-existent. There is also very little exploration of the problems and tensions of the inner city society; issues of access, equality and discrimination (East 1995) in general practice counselling services still receive too little attention.

As a result of a series of government initiatives focusing on the contribution primary care can make to community-based, preventive health care, general practitioners have already seen enormous changes to their working practices. In the new context of primary care groups as locality purchasers, yet working to national standards of quality and performance, there is a danger that counsellors in general practice, struggling to justify their existence, will lose sight of the social picture. However, another important government initiative, the setting up of a social exclusion unit in 1997, aims to address some of the most difficult problems facing society today, and to shift policy-making towards the prevention of social exclusion in six key areas:

- truancy
- school exclusion
- rough sleeping
- worst estates

- teenage parents
- sixteen to eighteen year olds.

It is significant that the unit is now seeking comments on deprived neighbourhoods struggling with the very problems brought by inner city patients, to do with class, culture, the uprooting of individuals and families from their homes and communities, as well as with other forms of social disruption or exclusion.

Nearly forty years ago, in 1957, Michael Balint was writing of urbanization, as a result of which 'a great number of people have lost their roots and connections, large families with their complicated and intimate interrelations tend to disappear, and the individual becomes more and more solitary, even lonely' (1964 p. 2). Now, in the late 1990s, counsellors in the inner city have much to offer by highlighting, alongside other forms of research, the different ways patients grapple with the problems of urbanization, and the value for them of finding a space in which their individual voices can be heard.

# 7

# Reflective practice and the postmodern context

*Marilyn Pietroni*

Here, too, the stage in Western culture and society that we are now entering – whether we see it as the third phase in Modernity, or as a new and distinctive 'post-modern' phase – obliges us to reappropriate values from renaissance humanism that were lost in the heyday of Modernity. Even at the core of 20th-century physics, idiosyncrasies of persons and cultures cannot be eliminated.

Stephen Toulmin, *Cosmopolis*

## SYNOPSIS

The working debates on counselling in general practice take place in a philosophical and historical context which affects how people think, how they speak and how they do things. This chapter aims to make that context more explicit, first by summarizing the philosophy of the reflective practice approach at Marylebone Health Centre and the University of Westminster department with which it is associated, and then by examining the current historical context.

A reflective practice approach aims to place in the foreground the complexity of real world problems brought by patients, and validates 'professional artistry', that artful yet technically-informed pragmatism that defines a practitioner's response (Schön 1991). Schön's now classic dictum of ensuring that relevance is sustained by linking 'the high ground' of academic and professional rigour with 'the swamp' of everyday practice is at the heart of this approach. Schön as a philosopher also legitimates indeterminacy, paradox and uniqueness as important features of professional practice (Schön 1983).

Historically, the work at Marylebone is taking place in a contemporary context which has been defined by social and cultural commentators as postmodern (Richards 1994, Parton 1994, Pietroni 1995, 1999, Rustin 1991). This perspective is examined here in order to create a critical context from which to examine the use of the technical term containment in the next chapter.

## REFLECTIVE PRACTICE: THE PHILOSOPHICAL CONTEXT

There are now numerous proponents of a reflective practice philosophy of which perhaps the best known are Schön (1987a), Kolb (1984) and Boud et al (1985). Some well-established critiques (Eraut 1995) and useful reviews of the literature (e.g. Atkins & Murphy 1993) also exist. Perhaps the most succinct summary of a reflective practice philosophy is a statement of Schön's thinking which can be found in his classic paper 'The crisis of professional knowledge and the pursuit of an epistemology of practice' (1992). Marylebone Health Centre and the Centre for Community Care and Primary Health at the University of Westminster have been particularly influenced by the work of Donald Schön who consulted to both academic and professional staff at critical stages in their development until his recent death.

Schön was one of the youngest ever Reith lecturers in 1970, who subsequently developed his thinking in the USA at the Massachusetts Institute of Technology over a period of more than thirty years. Separately and together with Chris Argyris, he examined over a lifetime the relationship between individual professionals and their organizational tasks. The foundation of their work dates back to two key conferences which were convened in the late 1960s and early 1970s to which a wide range of professionals were invited to discuss the current state and needs of professional knowledge and education. One profession after another described a crisis in professional knowledge which was epitomized by the gap between the academic rigour of professional training and research on the one hand and the messy, complex, indeterminate, and often unique problems found in everyday practice on the other.

From the conference data, Schön and his colleagues developed a model of four distinct professional types:

- the expert professional who claims expert knowledge which can sometimes result in being distanced from everyday problems
- the managerial professional who leaves behind her discipline of origin and assumes responsibility for planning, resource allocation and personnel
- the practical professional who takes a pragmatic, rational problem-solving approach, arriving at solutions by trial and error, and who is close to everyday problems
- the reflective practitioner who recognizes the limits of professional knowledge and action, then builds a cycle of action and reflection to maximize the capacity for critical thought, and produces a sense of professional freedom and connection with rather than distance from patients/clients/service users.

Obviously none of these categories occurs in a pure form but they provide a useful map with which to think about professionals and their knowledge (including theory) and action. In particular, the four categories signal the different ways professionals have found to manage the tensions between theory, practice and the management of scarce resources. At Marylebone Health Centre, the monthly sequence of lunchtime meetings described in Chapter 2 reflects our commitment to a continuous cycle of action and reflection on different aspects of the institutional task within a multi-professional and multi-agency context:

- the primary health care inter-agency perspective
- the process perspective: managing the impact, interactions and complexity of the work
- the academic perspective: use of theory and research evidence across professions
- the staff perspective: everyday practical management of systems and persons.

This sequence also ensures that the institutions of the health centre and of each professional sub-group within it are not allowed to become encapsulated like closed systems, but are required to remain, in a sense, uncomfortably-related across a series of differences which are continuously productive of thought.

This productive discomfort is in line with Schön's way of working. His further research was based on detailed individual analyses of examples of professional practice from a wide range of professions including architecture, music, psychoanalysis and engineering. The published examples are described in meticulous and subtle detail and Schön analyses in each a critical change in thinking that took place as the professional creatively adapted her initial 'high ground' perspective to the constraints of the everyday reality as a result of action and reflection (Schön 1987b). These are the shifts in perspective which he termed 'professional artistry' and which he considered to be usually unconscious but available for later explication. Mezirow (1981), in a much quoted paper on the aims of adult education, states that this kind of 'perspective transformation' is the key to advanced education, because it involves giving up the routinized habits that develop after basic training and fostering a continuous cycle of learning from complex experience.

Enid Balint, writing about the form of reflective supervision in general practice that has developed into the well-known Balint Group approach, described a reflective method remarkably close to Schön's own. She encouraged practitioners 'to speak freely without notes, contradict themselves if necessary, have second thoughts, remember things they thought they had forgotten; so that a complete picture emerged in which the feelings of the doctor himself [*sic*] were evident alongside the facts ....' (Elder & Samuel 1987, p. 96).

Like Schön, the Balints trusted the wisdom of the unconscious and of intuition as part of (rather than apart from) technical and theoretical rigour. Contradictions and ambiguities were seen by each as the vital place where rational consciousness and intuition meet and deep thought and learning have to begin. Schön's work on the reflective practice philosophy thus has close connections with well-established traditions in general practice and is summarized in Figure 7.1.

**Figure 7.1**   Summary of Schön's reflective practice philosophy (from Pietroni M 1993)

- A crisis in professional knowledge exists where the high ground of academic rigour and the lowland of messy practice do not connect.
- A form of professional artistry needs to be developed by stimulating living connections between theory, intuition and practice.
- Intuitive problem-solving needs to accompany hard knowledge and specific skills.
- Reflection-on-action and reflection-in-action (a 'double feedback loop') are vital to advanced practice.
- Innovative educational approaches are needed.

I have argued elsewhere that Schön's development of the reflective practice philosophy shares a common intellectual foundation with Bion's highly technical concept of containment as discussed in the next chapter (Pietroni M 1993). Both emphasize the centrality of 'attention and interpretation' when making sense of the communications of an individual or a group. Both emphasize that practitioners cannot and should not claim (like Schön's expert professional) 'to know' but need to retain (like his reflective practitioner) a sense of discovery in the present, an openness to surprise, an appreciation of the unfolding uniqueness of many of the problems which confront them and the constant modification required to pre-existent terms of reference (Bion 1965, 1970).

## IMPLICATIONS

The authors of this book owe much to this reflective practice philosophy, which has been largely responsible for our emphasis on direct and detailed clinical material with professional responses, changes of heart, dilemmas and mistakes openly revealed. Whilst on the one hand we are opening ourselves and our patients to greater scrutiny than a more summary form of clinical reportage would allow, on the other we hope to convey how complex this work is, how single models of counselling have little place in the general practice setting and how important are intuition, creative thinking and the unique attention and response given to each patient. Inevitably the material provided is still selected and abbreviated; it does not claim to be otherwise, but we hope that we have given enough of the mundane flows and discontinuities of the work for its burdensome complexity and frequent surprises to come through.

We have not neglected the 'high ground' in Schön's terms but in Part 3 have placed key knowledge and research evidence alongside the clinical material. This represents how the professional practitioner carries such knowledge in mind but can rarely apply it fully or neatly. Rather it informs and shapes thinking which is actually developed collaboratively between patient and professional or in the multi-professional team. Sometimes, as the clinical examples illustrate, it is necessary to make an exception, to put such thinking on one side and to go against the received wisdom of theory or research and do something that feels quite new or that does not fit into any particular model of counselling practice.

It is just such exceptions that provided the most interest for Schön in his world-wide 'on-the-spot' research workshops. Many of his students were professors themselves and he would invite them to talk about recent experiences in the workplace when something new or unexpected happened or when they did something they felt was 'wrong but right' or where someone felt stuck. He would then lead both individual and learning group through a series of tough questions that took them right to the heart of the reflective process, laying bare as he did so the layers of meaningless habit and ritual that stood in the way of recognizing the new. It could be an awesome process, for Schön somehow managed to combine the precision of the surgeon with the pragmatism of the home help. He was the master of this 'on-the-spot improvisation', an apt term which he chose to capture a peculiar blend of conscious and unconscious discovery drawn from the jazz which he so loved, and which, in Chapter 5, we have used as a metaphor for the rhythms of improvisation and routine in inner city counselling across the general practice year.

## THE HISTORICAL CONTEXT: A POSTMODERN SOCIETY?

The reflective practice philosophy outlined above has been generated by a particular social and historical context which Schön himself described as Beyond the Stable State (Schön 1971), now often described as postmodern (Rustin 1991, Hoggett 1992). Postmodernism offers a theoretical perspective with a set of illuminating core concepts that have been used in different ways in different fields, but about which there is some international consensus. These concepts have been drawn from a range of other theories, notably sociology and linguistics, and have been most frequently applied in the field of cultural studies. Because general practice, counselling and the multi-professional approach taken at Marylebone Health Centre occur within a western, capitalist culture at a particular point in history, the concepts of postmodernism help to illuminate the activities and their context in particular ways. Notably they help to draw together and make explicit some key features of the market approach to primary and community care introduced in the last ten years, which has increased the complexity of the overall field but of which counsellors working individually sometimes remain unaware.

Since the implementation of the NHS and Community Care Act 1990 (DoH 1990), costed episodes of care have been introduced into a health and community care service which had previously been poorly costed, audited and planned. General practitioners and their teams, already subject to new contractual legislation in lieu of their earlier freedoms, became part of a network of health and community services divided into different groups of purchasers and providers who were now required to establish contracts for service and payment within specified geographical cost centres. The change this so-called 'internal market' of care produced in the professional climate was as fundamental as when the NHS itself was established in 1948.

Quantification, prediction and planning became paramount and were accelerated by computer technology. A managerialist culture inevitably took over whilst professional values and practices came under fire. There were massive changes in the language used to describe professional practice at both micro (individual) and macro (local, regional or national) levels, so much so that glossaries were issued by many health and local authorities to help both professionals and service users adapt to the new and rapid changes in the naming and delivery of services.

Such changes are seen by writers on postmodernism as but one part of many wider changes in western society which have been taking place over the last fifty years (see Lyotard 1984, Jameson 1991). Disillusionment with radical politics and the socialist promise of the early twentieth century are said to have given way to a deeply uncertain world which accepts a relativist philosophy and the inevitable fragmentation of values, thought and beliefs that follows. This postmodern world is said to be characterized by a continuously dizzy pace of change with a consequent babble of languages (including professional language) and the erasure of familiar categories of thought and formal structures of all kinds. It is taken as given that knowledge is humanly constructed and expressed in arbitrary language which in turn leads to an unease with many forms of social authority. Most of all, however, Jameson's idea that we are facing 'the cultural logic of late capitalism' places an emphasis on deep and complex social patterns of which commodification, or the tendency to market everything and anything including health and community care, is fundamental (Jameson 1991).

In such a world, counselling in general practice is perhaps needed more than ever, but it is at risk as an activity because its evidence base is relatively weak and the expense in time, money and human resources is constantly challenged (Sibbald et al 1996b, Parry 1997). It is hard as a counsellor to be aware that one's client is at the same time not only the GP's patient but also a cost and a consumer in management's language, the language of the market. It is hard for both GPs and counsellors, absorbing as they do so much human distress every day, week and year, always to keep in mind the complex market context in which they now work, where employment structures, the financing of services and the very language they use can change at short notice. A summary of the core concepts of postmodernism with some examples of their application to the overall field of primary and community care is given in Figure 7.2 The application of these ideas to counselling in general practice is discussed in more detail by the author in a recent publication (Pietroni in Lees 1999).

## IN CONCLUSION ...

The patients we see as counsellors in an inner city general practice come from all over the world. It is truly a global city. A significant proportion come with extraordinary problems generated by horrific experiences in London or abroad. There are no 'easyfit' counselling approaches that we know of to meet the range of need with which we are confronted. That is why we have developed a menu of counselling services and use it flexibly but with rigorous scrutiny and debate.

Each patient is at the same time an NHS customer or consumer, a GP's patient and a counsellor's client and therefore simultaneously inhabits three domains of discourse: market, medical and psycho-social (Pietroni 1999). These three perspectives do not always cohere, and may actually conflict creating doubt about appropriate action. When in 1996 the counsellors at Marylebone Health Centre decided to remain part of the 'care culture' of general practice and not merely of the 'cure culture', some liberation followed from an outcome-driven approach but justification in terms of the market model and an evidence base also has to be found.

The menu of counselling services went some way to rationing resources as stringently as possible and allowed more patients to be seen and wastage to be minimized. However, the term 'menu' is itself a hybrid generated by a postmodern consumerist world where odd new language sets arise with local meanings and have little impact on counselling training courses or the debates that surround them.

The next chapter will try to address some of the complexity of putting a reflective practice approach into action in this kind of historical context by selecting one concept, containment, and following it through from the academic high ground of its abstract definitions to the swamp of its contradictory meanings-in-use in multi-professional practice.

**Figure 7.2**   Core concepts of postmodernism (reprinted with permission from Lees 1999/Routledge)

**Commodification and the global market**
- Turning everything (including care) into tradeable commodities
- Community Care Market News: the share price gazette of home and residential care services published by Laing and Buisson with column headings such as 'Forensic mental health a niche market'
- Commissioning of care and the contract culture; international homecare agencies
- The purchaser/provider split and associated change to the language of the market
- Emphasis on cost volume and specified outcomes or products; short term output; time-based and tariff-based services e.g.: clinical 'episodes' or 'packages' of care, and referrals to secondary care services
- Expanding international market in independent consultancies, information networks, and health and social care provision

**Complexification in relation to critical change**
- Fundamental changes in health and community care policy, philosophy and organization: repeated reorganizations and rewriting of job and person specifications, rewriting job titles, reselections of staff
- Mixture of clinical and market criteria in frontline and managerial decision making
- Increased inter-agency and inter-sector collaboration bringing a 'jangle of jargons'
- Increased complaints promoted by consumer charters
- Complex relations with a wide range of information technology via audit, quality and performance measures
- Versatility on the frontline required by the cultural melting pot of the inner cities
- Breakdown in family structures and increased poverty and mobility
- Ideologies of political correctness: a persecutory culture which inhibits debate and is intolerant of differences of view, values and language
- The contested nature of the concept of normalcy at a time of high profile normalisation policies e.g. in fields of mental health, disability, learning difficulties, homelessness, parenting etc.

**The global city and a new medievalism (Eco 1987)**
- Fundamentalist conflicts across racial, religious, political and ideological groups
- Increased violence at work, at home, in cars and on the street
- Extreme distress of refugees and torture victims from across the world present in general practice
- The illicit drugs market and associated baronial sub-culture
- International client/patient/refugee populations make distant wars local e.g. Bosnian/Serb conflicts, torture victims etc.
- Language and interpretation issues confound communication
- Cultural differences saturate everyday practice e.g. female circumcision, gender roles, marital and ownership conventions

**Crisis in authority and leadership**
- Conflicts between managerialist and professionalist values and approaches in all agencies; rise of anti-professional lobbies and young supermarket style management
- Clumsy restructuring: dismantling of old centres of excellence, closure of newly commissioned units, severe shortages of basic facilities e.g. inpatient beds, home aids and equipment
- Privileged new generation of non-professional manager/leaders with high tech skills and denigration of old-style experienced clinician
- Increase in early retirements and redundancy packages leading to rapidly changing leaders and leadership systems in clinical practice and academia

**Figure 7.2**   Core concepts of postmodernism (*cont'd*)

- Cost, volume and output-led decision making competes with clinically-led decision making
- Recruitment problems in nursing, social work and general practice

**Superficial language games: a crisis in meaning and representation**
- Contested terms: patient, client, consumer, user; counsellor, counselling psychologist, psychotherapist; needs-led assessment, user-centredness, eligibility criteria, care management; increased choice; quality measures and performance indicators
- Care in the community as a term for unplanned and under resourced de-institutionalization
- Philosophy and language of partnership in conflict of interest situations e.g. child protection, mental health, care of elders
- Policy taboo on the individualized recording of unmet need at needs assessment stage of care management in social services
- 'Acronymitis': the ubiquitous use of acronyms as a social defence against rapid change to give an illusion of being up-to-date by knowing the latest new service, research or educational consortia or theoretical perspective

**Banalization and dumbing down: a superficial amalgam of sentimentality, parody and pastiche**
- Buzz words with a hollow public relations quality: user-centredness, seamless service, quality, joined-up thinking
- Bizarre new jargon: social bathing, health bathing, qualy (quality of life years)
- Buzz phrases that normalize radical and untested ideas: the market of care, the 'mixed welfare economy'
- Simplistic colour matching of client and practitioner e.g. fostering and adoption, ignoring race, ethnicity and religion
- Homogenization through procedures that silently blend clinical and cost issues: needs assessment, care packages, care plans, which really mean eligibility tests and rationing criteria
- The title key worker: often applied to part-timers or others low in power and status in the multi-professional/multi-agency team
- Partnership policies in conflicted areas of practice that promote fudged compromises and undermine independent critical thinking and the professional assessment of individuals

**Impact of new technology and rapid information exchange**
- Challenges to confidentiality from inter-agency databases and collaboration
- Reception desks: interaction with computers competes with, and often supersedes, interaction with human beings in hospitals and general practice
- Improved information provides opportunity for regulated, targeted innovations e.g. care episodes, home bathing services, home repairs, putting-to-bed services
- Audit and information systems associated with the purchaser/provider split and the monitoring of service contracts introduces annual regulatory changes and associated instability in the workplace
- Increased time has to be allocated to audit and performance review
- Life and life styles mimic technology e.g. internet romance and adultery; technological pets: fashion and homestyles follow film fads: short contacts replace relationships in a 'delete-open-new-file-retitle-rewrite' cycle

# 8

# Theory in use: perspectives on containment

*Marilyn Pietroni*

Great joy is had in the endless invention of turns of phrase, of words and meanings, the process behind the evolution of language on the level of *parole*. But undoubtedly even this pleasure depends on a feeling of success won at the expense of an adversary – at least one adversary, and a formidable one: the accepted language, or connotation […] the observable social bond is made of language moves.

Jean-François Lyotard, *The postmodern condition*

## SYNOPSIS

This chapter selects the term containment as a vehicle for an exploration which starts on the conceptual high ground and then moves to what Schön called the 'swamp' of frontline practice. Conceptual and practical links are suggested between Bion's concept of containment (1962) and the Balints' 'flash' technique, the former being more familiar to counsellors, especially if psychodynamically trained, and the latter to GPs (Balint E & Norell 1973).

The concept of containment was selected as a starting point because of its widespread use and relevance to different kinds of work in the general practice setting and its frequent application to work with individuals, teams and networks. The concept is sufficiently elastic to be applied to one-to-one work between patients and GPs, counsellors or complementary therapists and to a multi-professional teamwork process.

The exploration of the concept in use at Marylebone Health Centre is complicated by the multi-professional nature of the team and their wide range of belief systems and language groups. In the process of two years of detailed 'reflection on action' in the monthly academic meetings, the team had to cope with their discovery that the term containment was being used in contradictory ways. They decided a new and more grounded definition in shared and ordinary (non-professional) language was needed, if the term was to become a vehicle for inter-professional collaboration and if unhelpful, anti-task social defences were to be minimized.

## FROM HIGH GROUND TO SWAMP

The chapter begins with a brief exploration of the psychodynamic meaning of containment which though complex has been opened up by some useful commentaries (Meltzer 1978, Moustaki 1981, Hinshelwood 1989, Symington & Symington 1996). Counsellors with a psychodynamic orientation will be familiar with the origins and meaning of the term which has frequently been applied in the worlds of counselling, psychotherapy and family therapy, following its development in the psychoanalytic world in the 1950s (e.g. Box et al 1981, Wiener & Sher 1998). Hopefully, other members of the primary health care team less familiar or enamoured with the psychodynamic literature will find this bird's eye view of the concept useful, not least because the argument will move from the psychoanalytic origins of the term to its varied use in the more eclectic culture of the multi-professional team.

A link is made between the original specialist definition of containment usually attributed to Bion (1959), and the development of the idea of the 'flash' technique in the work of Enid and Michael Balint, which is very familiar to most general practitioners. Like Bion, both were psychoanalysts, and their concept of something communicated in a brief general practice consultation in a disorganized way suddenly becoming crystallized, understood and available for examination, has some common features with Bion's concept of containment, where something communicated unconsciously, and often beyond words, emerges into consciousness (Balint & Norell 1973).

The chapter will move on, in Schön's terms (1987a or b), from this theoretical high ground to the swamp of everyday practice, by examining the range of rather different meanings-in-use for the term containment, discovered in two years of multi-professional debate in the monthly Marylebone Health Centre academic meetings. This part of the chapter shows how a sophisticated concept developed in a specialist setting can and has been adapted to a generalist one, where a range of different philosophical, theoretical and clinical models necessarily co-exist. This adaptation is not seen as a form of 'dumbing down'. Rather, an examination of the different meanings actually in use is seen as an important reflective exercise, if a multi-professional team is to develop the capacity to work inter-professionally with the kinds of problems that are thrown up by life in a capital city. Too often such a team can hide behind different professional languages in which the same word is used without awareness that it means something quite different to different members and has quite different practical implications. It would have been easier, for example, to write this book about counselling concentrating only on our own use of the term without reference to the contradictory uses in the team as a whole. Instead we start with our own perspective and then trace it through the somewhat unsettling multi-professional debate and surprising discoveries that were made in the academic meetings.

## CONTAINMENT OF THE PSYCHE-SOMA: THE PSYCHOANALYTIC ORIGINS OF THE TERM

Containment is not an easy concept to understand or to put into practice. However, thanks to the work of Hinshelwood (1989), it is now possible to identify the origins of selected psychoanalytic concepts fairly easily. He has done a wonderful job of defining concepts and mapping the development of their different meanings across a range of primary and secondary sources. Hinshelwood describes containment as a 'decisive concept' and points out its close links to Melanie Klein's concept of projective identification 'in which one person in some sense contains a part of another' (p. 246). He chooses a quotation from the psychoanalyst Rosenfeld to show the developing relationship between these two terms, a quotation which is illuminating from the point of view of general practice, because it refers implicitly to physical as well as mental experience, and it is often the body that patients bring first to the GP as the container of the symptom of their inner disease.

The patient ... showed that he had projected his *damaged* self containing the *destroyed* world, not only *into* all the other patients, but into me, and had changed me in this way. But instead of becoming relieved by this projection he became more anxious, because he was afraid of what I was *putting back into him*, whereupon his introjective processes became severely disturbed. (Rosenfeld 1952, pp. 80–81, quoted in Hinshelwood 1989, p. 244 emphasis added)

The words 'damaged', 'destroyed', 'into' and 'putting back into him', convey a physicality behind their abstraction that allows one to imagine, in a kind of shadow play alongside the adult verbal exchanges, the mime-like movements of a child's sometimes violent interaction with another. What the quotation makes clear is that containment is a powerfully felt active and interactive process which involves a process of shedding and projecting what are felt to be damaged, frightening or unwanted parts of the self for psycho-somatic containment inside another.

Freud had written many years previously that the ego which mediates between different levels of consciousness (within and between individuals) is in the first instance a body ego: 'The ego is ultimately derived from bodily sensations, chiefly from those springing from the surface of the body.' (Freud 1923 p. 26) He explained the relationship between sense perceptions which have their origins in the body (hearing, sight, touch, taste, smell), mental images (which he considered to be primitive, 'Thinking in pictures is ... only a very incomplete form of thought' p. 21) and words.

Thus he laid the ground for Bion's work on container/contained which discriminates between communication where emotional life and depth can be tolerated, however confused, violent or inarticulate, and communication which is hollow or emotionally empty, or uses dissociated physical signs, where the emotional links between thoughts, words and psyche-soma have been unconsciously severed. Hinshelwood summarizes Bion's view of these vital links as follows: 'Thus putting experiences into thoughts and thoughts into words, entails a repeated chain of linking processes modelled on physical intercourse between two bodily parts' (Hinshelwood 1991, p. 341).

## The container contained relationship

Bion defines containment in terms of a shifting container/contained relationship (1962). The concept is based on the model of the mother as a container for the infant's projected needs, feelings and unwanted parts. A defining feature of what has to be contained is that either it has not reached a verbal state, or it has burst open the capacity of words to contain meaning. Bion gives the example of the stammer where emotion disrupts the containing forms of words and grammar. The containing other receives this pre-verbal raw material and is then involved in a reflective psycho-somatic process in which psychic digestion takes place alongside disciplined physical awareness. Therefore the process of understanding what is being contained requires emotional labour of a profound psychosomatic kind and is not simply sitting and listening, important though that is.

The concept of containment, or the container/contained relation, depends heavily on two other linked concepts which are technical and also somewhat difficult to understand, namely projective and introjective identification (Klein 1946). Rosenfeld's quotation cited above shows these interactive processes of identification at work. The patient tries to get rid of some unwanted, uncomfortable, damaged part of himself by projecting it into another (or others) using the mechanism of projective identification. The 'psycho-somatic stuff projected by the patient for containment into the inner space of the containing other is often somatically felt before it is psychically recognized. Indeed, it may not actually be psychically recognized and may remain pre-conscious for some time. Either way, the process of containing such inchoate, primitive material is referred to as introjective identification. Something has been overtly or covertly pushed into the container who now carries and is changed by it. The container's powers of observation, reflection and discriminating thought determine to what extent the projected and unwanted part of the self can later become consciously articulated and reintegrated.

Containing can therefore be likened to a process of psychic digestion in which the container's senses first receive and examine (chew over) what has been projected before the next stage can begin: the emotional and cognitive work of separating what was felt to be mental poison or waste matter from what is psychologically useful and needs to be reintegrated by the originator. Then a new stage of 'making sense', or articulating what was previously inchoate, can begin. The containment process is somewhat paradoxical: precise and disciplined on the one hand, chaotic and confusing on the other.

Bion uses the term *reverie* to describe the calm and receptive state of mind required of the containing other who is ready to introject and make sense of what has been projected (1962). The container in a state of reverie identifies at a primitive psycho-somatic level with the 'undifferentiated stuff' that has been taken in and only then begins to sift and try to understand it, before going on to detoxify the more alarming aspects and eventually finding a safe enough means of expression. This process eventually allows the modified contents to be returned in a safer and more tolerable form.

The model provided by the container of not only surviving the process of containing such hazardous stuff, but also being able to distil and return it as something useful, offers a model of the container/contained relationship that can itself be introjected. In the future, a reservoir of repeated experiences of self-containment strengthens inner resources sufficiently for them to be drawn upon repeatedly, even under duress. The active container contained relation provides a model for continuing personal development.

The prototypical psycho-somatic origins of the model are described by Bion as the mother and infant, or more primitively, the nipple and breast, penis and vagina, and it is to these prototypes that Hinshelwood is referring when he uses the term 'physical intercourse' as quoted above. This movement in description in the literature between body metaphors and mind metaphors reflects the complexity not only of the concept of containment and therefore the relation between container and contained, but also of the living relation between body and mind, a relation which is central to the task of understanding that faces practitioners with each new patient, especially in the general practice setting where patients usually present with a physical sign in the first instance. When a patient like the Torture Victim in Chapter 11 is referred to the counselling service, or the Refugee Artist in Chapter 9 who is struggling for mental life in the face of heavy anti-psychotic medication, or the Uprooted Schoolgirl in Chapter 12 caught between languages, it is not unusual for the main means of communication to be through projective identification with little use of words. The quality of containment provided by the counsellor is then vital to the patient's mental survival and development.

## CONTAINMENT IN THE GENERAL PRACTICE SETTING: LINKS WITH BALINT'S 'FLASH' TECHNIQUE

The concept of containment reviewed above derives originally from the theory and practice of psychoanalysis. As a concept related to practice technique, it is usually familiar to counsellors trained psychodynamically. Although GPs train differently, they have their own historical links with psychoanalytic thinking, some of which may be unfamiliar to counsellors. As one might expect, the rather different terms used reflect the economy of response expected of a GP in a brief consultation, but on closer examination the ideas have much in common.

The nature of the GP/patient consultation was looked at in depth, drawing on a psychoanalytic perspective, by Michael and Enid Balint (Balint 1964, Balint & Norell 1973). For many years, GPs met in 'Balint seminars' at the Tavistock Clinic and elsewhere, presenting their cases for discussion with a psychoanalyst or psychoanalytical psychotherapist to examine in depth the unconscious aspects of the doctor/patient relationship.

Balint drew on this work when he described the flash technique which, though quite different in some respects from Bion's concept of containment, is similar in others, especially in terms of the quality of listening required (Bion's reverie) and its paradoxical combination of freedom and discipline. The 'flash' technique moves away from the traditional aim of 'pinpointing the seat of the trouble' to an alternative aim of 'providing the patient with the opportunity to communicate whatever it is s/he wants' in a 'brief, intense and close contact' and following up on what has been communicated at a subsequent meeting (Balint & Norell 1973 p. xi). The moment of the flash is that moment when communication is successful and the doctor has been able to hear, to sense and to think about what is being communicated in such a way that a shared moment of understanding occurs that allows what follows to have an emotionally substantial quality, sometimes with and sometimes without practical implications.

Enid Balint, describing how to develop the liberation of the 'flash' technique described three working principles:

1. The doctor should not be TOO preoccupied with theories or preconceived questions.
2. The doctor needs to consider what to do with his/her observations.
3. The doctor needs to respect the patient's right to hide or not disclose his/her secrets.

In her development of these principles, the links between the 'flash' technique (familiar to GPs) and the use of containment (usually familiar to counsellors) becomes more evident. Both depend on that quality of listening, described by Bion as reverie, that allows clarification of meaning to emerge from both unconscious and conscious sources, and is often registered psycho-somatically. Enid Balint's chapter '*The flash technique: its freedom and discipline*' suggests further links between these two important concepts (see Figure 8.1).

> **Figure 8.1**   The Balint's 'flash' technique: links with Bion's containment (from Balint & Norell 1973, p. 20)
>
> If one has a theory, one is limited by the theory; if one has not theory, it is difficult to observe [. .] but it gives freedom to observe. This freedom is only useful if it is coupled with discipline: in our case the discipline of careful and attentive observations, and the ability to know how much of what is observed originated with the patient and how much is contributed by the doctor him/herself [...]
>    The difficulty is more in keeping up the intensity of attentive observation after a decision has been made to comment or interpret [...] The doctor has to reflect silently about his observations and their meaning: identify with the patient, develop ideas about him, and then to intervene by making a comment or interpretation to test out his line of thought. As we know, the silent reflecting part of the process is done very rapidly.

# IMPLICATIONS FOR PRACTICE
## Awareness of social defences

If a practitioner can use these abstract ideas about how to listen and how to think about what a patient is communicating, it does not necessarily mean that s/he 'gets it right'. Nevertheless, it does help the work in an important way. Pamela Smith writes of 'the emotional labour' required of professionals if they are to combat the worst forms of stress arising from their work in ways that do not involve developing a thick defensive skin (Smith 1992).

Often professionals build up a defence against the repeated pain, frustration, helplessness and intimacy that confronts them in their work as a way of surviving and this is encouraged in basic training as part of establishing the appropriate distance of a boundaried professional identity. GPs, counsellors and complementary therapists, for instance, engage with the most private aspects of either the bodies or the minds of their patients and sometimes both. They and their patients need help in managing this intimacy from a mutually understood repertoire of role behaviours which involve different kinds of distance regulation.

Professional distance is necessary but it can be overdone. It can become a kind of protective habit worn to convey confidence and purity, to conceal uncertainty, to impart a false sense of expert knowledge or, most important of all, to establish and sustain membership of a professional tribe with its hierarchical internal class system. Here, Schön's distinction between the expert practitioner, who assumes expert knowledge and establishes distance from the client, and the reflective practitioner, who recognizes the limits of professional knowledge and establishes a sense of partnership and connection with the client in a joint exploration, is relevant.

The attempt to contain a range of often disturbing psycho-somatic communications in a brief period of time therefore involves a tension between the distance required to allow productive reflection to occur, and the intimacy needed to be available and useful as a container. Isabel Menzies Lyth's classic article (1988) describes the social defence systems used by a nursing hierarchy in a teaching hospital. She shows only too clearly what happens if the anxiety about letting something disturbing in is allowed to generate a defensive social system based primarily on distance: staff morale drops, sickness rates increase and attention is displaced onto organizational rituals which are of minor importance whilst the real nursing tasks are neglected. So too it can be in general practice, whether one is a doctor, counsellor, receptionist or complementary therapist. A defensive thick skin can be created that inhibits the capacity of the individual professional to think independently and to use initiative and imagination. The thick skin also ensures that the patient's communications bounce off rather than being taken in, thought about and responded to appropriately.

When in the next section we turn from theory to practice, it becomes clearer just how such social defences find expression and how contested the idea of containment really is. When the members of the multi-professional team were given the space to struggle openly with the meaning of the term containment (and therefore with this tension between distance and intimacy) they discovered they were using it in different and contradictory ways.

## Containment of the psyche-soma: an exploration of meanings-in-use in the multi-professional team

When Marylebone Health Centre staff spent six of their monthly academic meetings examining what was meant by the much-used term containment by different members of the interprofessional team, it became clear that there were almost as many meanings-in-use as there were members in the team.

The counsellors used the term in much the way outlined above, as originally defined by Bion, meaning that some kind of useful transformation was felt to be possible if a difficult (confused, painful, violent, inarticulate) communication could be taken in, 'chewed over', detoxified and handed back in a recognizable and more bearable form, making it available internally for future use.

The GPs used the term containment frequently but rarely meant the same as the counsellors. More often they meant they could do little for a patient with either medical treatment or advice, so what was possible was simply to provide some kind of support or safety net.

When the complementary practitioners used the term they tended to mean something similar to the GPs. Occasionally, however, GPs and complementary practitioners would mean something different again by the term, more akin to control or repression, for example when a patient was seriously problematic and in frequent contact with the practice in a rather demanding and difficult way that took resources from more needy patients.

The discovery of this range of three different meanings-in-use for the term containment (transformative, safety net and repressive) led to a decision to use one year of the lunchtime academic meetings (about 8 hours after holidays) looking at examples of use by the multi-professional team and generating some differentiated but shared meanings in the language of everyday speech that we could all understand and use. The choice of a shared common language was important because each profession had its own jargon or technical language that seemed to obscure differences in meaning and to impede inter-professional communication in the team.

This first year cycle of academic meetings was an example of reflection on action; in Schön's terms the first cycle allows change and reframing to occur within a single, relatively simple system by reflection after practice. The second cycle of reflection he called 'reflection-in-action' which is more complex. First, it takes place in the midst of practice pressures and not with hindsight; second, it needs to combine intuition, intellect and professional judgement in some kind of on-the-spot experiment or improvisation which goes against the grain of well-worn ritual and modifies basic assumptions, the apparent 'givens' of everyday practice and organizational life.

A second year of academic meetings was therefore later devoted to applying and testing the new shared meanings on further practice examples in each of the different professional units. This decision allowed the second cycle of reflection-in-action to occur, and provided the opportunity for promoting real organizational learning (Argyris & Schön 1978).

Figure 8.2 contains the three definitions that were agreed at the end of this work. This is followed by a brief explanation of how the team found they were using these definitions after a further year's work.

### Transformative containment

This meaning is the most complex and was used by all members of the multi-professional team but perhaps most commonly by the counsellors. As described above, it has been substantially theorized by Bion (1962). After discussion the descriptive term transformative was selected because all professions in the team could identify with the word and the idea, notwithstanding their different world views and theoretical orientations. The meaning was finally restated as in Figure 8.2.

The most common use of this meaning of the term was with those patients where the GPs or complementary therapists could make a relatively quick assessment, perhaps drawing on Balint's flash technique, followed by some useful therapeutic intervention, or where the counsellors had a patient referred with whom they could do some constructive brief work that was likely to achieve some form of limited transformation. Most, but not all, of the stories of patients in counselling in Part 3 of this book fall into this category of meaning.

---

**Figure 8.2**   The meanings-in-use of containment at Marylebone Health Centre

1. Transformative: This patient seems to want to understand their symptoms/difficulties/behaviour and to grow/change their lifestyle/behaviour; furthermore we think that with our help they can do so, at least to some extent. Therefore we will take in their communication in some depth, try to understand it, and perhaps begin to help to articulate it. In the process, we will take some of the sting out of the needs and communication they are bringing to us, so that it feels safer to take them back in a newly-integrated way.

2. Safety net: We probably cannot help this patient to become much healthier, or to learn or to grow, but we can help him/her, or his/her situation, not to deteriorate by being available, listening, and offering treatment, support, advice or clarification when needed. The problem is that the patient is motivated, but for a variety of reasons (the state of our skills and knowledge, the nature of the illness or behaviour or a lack of resources), we can help only a little and mainly in a supportive way.

3. Repressive: This patient seems constantly to be seeking help, often across a range of services in and outside of the practice, and often in a way that eventually wastes resources and upsets staff. By the nature of their difficulties there is very little that we can do to help, but we need to limit the wastage of resources and the damaging impact that the patient's behaviour is having on staff. Understanding or intervening does not seem to help, the pattern of contact just endlessly repeats itself, so we have to take firm control.

---

## Safety net containment

The most common use of this meaning of the term was in relation to long term seriously ill patients with severe or chronic physical illness such as heart disease, cancer or multiple sclerosis; or with severe mental or neurological illness such as schizophrenia, dementia, severe and recurrent depression or bipolar affective disorder. From the restated meaning, it was clear that some elements of Bion's definition of the term remained. There is a recognition that a particular quality of listening and thinking makes an important contribution to the continuing care of the patient, even if it cannot contribute in a curative way. There is also the recognition that the resource framework of the NHS cannot stretch to provide as much of this type of containment as the patient might feel is wanted or needed or the worker may wish to provide.

## Repressive containment

This meaning was the most contentious. All professions recognized that there were times when they had to set exceptional limits on their interactions with patients in a way that could feel brutal. On the one hand they recognized that this was part of being a professional, maintaining appropriate distance and being clear about what was and was not possible; on the other hand, there was a quality about this form of containment that made them feel uncomfortable, frustrated and often guilty no matter how much they tried to understand the process at work. In part this was the effect of the patient powerfully transferring his sense of responsibility for himself on to the practitioner concerned, sometimes with the covert blessing of another member of the team. Often, this would happen between the GPs and the massage therapists to whom patients might be referred when the GP needed a break from the pressure. Usually however, this form of containment was used because the professional or the practice as a whole had been 'run dry' by a patient who seemed unable to take anything in but repeatedly came back for more like an insatiable baby.

## IN CONCLUSION . . .

The gap between theory and practice identified by Schön was rediscovered at Marylebone Health Centre as a result of this exercise. The team discussions were carried out in the reflective practice tradition and brought many shocks, some of them painful to us, but achieved the following important outcomes:

- Multi-professional or parallel working changed to inter-professional collaboration based on a deeper understanding of differences and explicit commonalities.
- Professional jargon was reduced so that more accurate communication between professionals could occur.
- Social defences were identified and some of their harmful effects on the professionals and their practice were reduced (less professional isolation, reduced guilt, improved team support, clearer limits, more thoughtful responses to patients' needs, fewer 'heartsink' patients created by professionals being unable to say no).
- A shared recognition of the institutional task of inner city general practice with its finite resources was established; idealism, guilt and cynicism gave way to a greater realism.

Each different type of containment defined in this work has a place in the services which inner city general practice can provide. The clinical examples in this book will illustrate each of these meanings in use. Our aspiration is naturally to offer as much of a transformative approach as possible, whilst the reality is that only about one third of the activities in general practice are transformative, one third are to do with sustaining the status quo and preventing deterioration, and one third are to do with managing an individual or family situation which is deteriorating and will go on doing so whatever interventions are made.

# Practice: inside counselling in the inner city

based on the stories of six patients who received counselling at Marylebone Health Centre

## Introduction

Then I heard an alternative way of presenting clinical material which seemed to address the fundamental dynamic of the 'case presentation' itself [...] The patient was allowed to occupy a quite different place in the clinical discourse and the audience perceived the material and the analytic situation in a new light. The patient ceased being an object and became in some measure a subject – not so unlike the audience who were listening to his [*sic*] story.

Ivan Ward, *The presentation of case material in clinical discourse*

Part 3 is written, as far as possible, in the words of those who are involved in the system of counselling in general practice. The setting, as we have shown in Part 1, is quite unlike private practice or a single profession counselling agency to which GPs refer. For example, with our first patient, described in Chapter 9, those involved included two GPs, the counsellor, two practice nurses, a community psychiatric nurse, a consultant psychiatrist and two receptionists and last but not least the patient herself. With others there is simply one GP, the receptionists and the counsellor, but even then the situation is far from simple because the patient may or may not know the receptionists well, and may have a long contact with the GP dating back over several years, whereas the counsellor may be providing only a few sessions. These contextual factors affect the meaning and significance of the counselling for the patient, which may be only one part of an overall picture of what is provided at the health centre and elsewhere.

It has not been possible to reflect the chronology of the work in the stories that follow. This would have taken too long and been somewhat laboured. However, in each story the sequence of what happens can usually be inferred from the different perspectives of those involved. We have included ambiguities and contradictions where these were a real part of what occurred. The purpose of leaving in such inconsistencies is to avoid an artificial orderliness, and to show the context and content of counselling in general practice in all its complexity. Our aim has been to demonstrate that important and sometimes contradictory dialogues, with different members of the team, can occur piecemeal and in parallel, and that this is in the nature of work in the setting of inner city general practice. In all stories key facts have been changed to protect confidentiality.

The research interviews undertaken for this book sometimes revealed significant relationships of which we, as counsellors, were not previously aware, for example with the receptionists and practice nurses. We take the view that this is likely often to be the case, however hard the team works on communication, since the counsellors are usually only at the practice one day a week, and the multi-professional team only meets once a week. For these reasons, although it is important to value the counselling relationship as a rare and special opportunity for patients to have that 'still point' in the practice, when they can think and talk within a clear time and space, it is also important not to allow that positive sense of something precious to turn into something more narcissistic. Counselling should not be something mystifying, secretive or inexplicable to others, and should rather be simply one part of the patient's ordinary experience of what the practice provides. Good general practice counselling, in our view, usually needs to have that mundane quality to help the work become integrated into the patient's everyday life.

# 9

# The refugee artist

*Marilyn Pietroni*

For surely it is one of the unhappiest characteristics of the age to have produced more refugees, migrants, displaced persons, and exiles than ever before in history, most of them as an accompaniment and ironically enough, as afterthoughts of great post-colonial and imperial conflicts.

Edward Saïd, *Culture and Imperialism*

## SYNOPSIS

This story covers the period between March 1993 and the present time. The patient has been seen by the counsellor about forty times, at about six weekly intervals (Service D: intermittent) with longer breaks over holidays. The pattern was changed briefly to weekly sessions (Service B: brief work) at a time of crisis. The patient sees the GP and practice nurses on a regular basis for medication and becomes a client of the community mental health team (CMHT). Thinking about this patient's long term needs helped the counselling team to refine the Menu of Counselling Services that was being developed throughout this period, particularly Service D (intermittent).

The story tells, in the patient's own words, what it is like to be a refugee with severe mental health problems in the inner city. The counsellor and other members of the multi-professional team and inter-agency network tell of the remarkably creative relationships she builds with them. They worked hard to provide containment, mostly of the safety net variety which sometimes became transformative.

A balance has been sought here, between a chronological narrative and a focus on three critical periods, starting with the referral. The term patient is used to avoid the clumsy patient/client and, as with all the stories, key facts have been changed to protect confidentiality.

## EARLY WORK

### The first GP's story (1993)

*Origins of the referral*

Miriana first came to this country as a refugee from Romania about eight years ago when … homeless and deeply distressed … she was given bed and breakfast accommodation in one of the hotels in our patch …. She told me she'd been in mental hospital in Romania after hearing voices and so on and told me what anti-psychotic medication she'd been on … so I put her on the UK version and she seems to have ticked over alright until recently. Now she's more settled … she wants more out of life and I think she's right … I'm ready to reduce her medication if I thought she could be monitored and supported while I'm doing it … I wonder if you counsellors would touch this one?

*The referral form*

Miriana Pilescu, age 44, diagnosed schizophrenic/manic depressive psychosis. Several psychiatric hospital admissions (Romania). Refugee in B&B. Lives alone. Depressed and wants to talk to someone. Can you help? Can we discuss?

Medication: Modecate depot injections 25 mg 3 weekly. Lithium Carbonate 1200 mg a day. Melleril 100 mg a day.

Other practitioners: none at present.

*The GP placed the form in the counsellors' referral folder on Friday for collection the following Wednesday when the counsellor is next at the practice.*

### The counsellor's story (1993)

*Receiving the referral*

As a part-timer I'm only in on one day a week, Wednesdays …. I depend on suitable, clear referrals because my aim (and the GP's wish) is that most of my time should be spent seeing patients … the practice's audit is based on the numbers of patients we see … and we have to satisfy the health authority and the practice that we are worth our money …. On receiving this referral form, I wondered what Dr Thomas was up to … she knows the research on counselling and brief psychotherapy …. She knows only too well that brief counselling (*in 1993, before the Menu of Services was introduced, all we were offering at the health centre*) is unlikely to be all that helpful to someone with a severe mental illness … who really needs long term support from the community mental health team ….

It feels like an inappropriate referral … and I have three other refer-rals this week to deal with … in my admin half hour … next week the doctors will be asking why we never have any vacancies. How can we clear the waiting list if they refer patients like this and we agree to see them? I must discuss with Dr Thomas ….

### Discussing the referral

*A discussion takes place between GP and counsellor in which Dr Thomas makes it clear that she knows only too well that Miriana does not look like an appropriate referral but there was 'something about her'. Though aware that the counsellors now have a waiting list, Dr Thomas did not change her view because she felt there was something exceptional about this patient. The coun-sellor agrees, after some debate, to an assessment only (this was before the introduction of the Patient Request Form).*

## Counsellor's story continued

I agree to see and assess the patient but tell myself I need my brains tested … I seem to be ignoring all that I know and simply following my gut feeling … based of course on the effect Miriana has already had on Dr Thomas …. I remind myself that the GPs are often too optimistic … and send an appointment for two weeks later, my first vacancy.

### The first appointment

I'm surprised to find a well-dressed, tall and attractive woman waiting for me in the waiting room … but there is something depressed about her as well … and her hair's a bit wild …. Why am I surprised that she looks so good? Is this a prejudice against mentally ill people which I thought I'd abandoned long ago … or is this Miriana's paradox? ….

I'm momentarily shocked to find I have these thoughts and try unsuccessfully to unscramble whether they are prejudice, clinical judgement or counter-transference as I walk along the corridor with Miriana and prepare to listen to her story …. I must clear my mind before I get there …. I'm aware of trying to put this debate which I can't answer 'on hold' so I can clear the surface of my mind and be ready to listen properly … not a good start … here goes ….

As Miriana sits down, I explain that I understand she has told her doctor that she wants to talk to someone … as I'm the counsellor in the practice … Dr Thomas thought I might be of some use …. I add that I however don't know if I can be … but we can try and find out today if possible …. Perhaps Miriana can tell me what she had in mind? I say that we have about forty five minutes left today ….

Miriana sat back in her seat and appeared to relax but I noticed her shoulders were tense and rather hunched over ... she did indeed have an atmosphere of depression about her ... her eyes were drawn she looked tired ... even exhausted. Hardly surprising, I thought, with all that medication inside her .... I soon found myself wondering as she told her story, what she would be like without so much medication ....

## The patient's story (1993)

Mrs Pietroni ... (can I call you that?) ... I am very depressed. My life is terrible, truly terrible .... I do nothing but sleep .... I can't stop sleeping and it makes it impossible for me to do my work .... My work is very important to me .... Really I am an artist, I trained as an artist, but I can never do my painting because I'm always sleeping .... I can't get up in the morning ... it's lunch time before I can do anything .... Then after I have had something to eat, I just fall asleep again in the chair .... I live a useless life .... I hate this life .... I am an artist and I want to paint ... but how can I when I feel like this?

*As she speaks she leans forward and seems to try and get the message into my body as well as my mind in an urgent way ... but there is a trailing off ... as if helplessness inevitably gets the better of her ....*

*I say that Dr Thomas explained that she's on some medication and that it was given to her in the past when she had a breakdown .... I ask if she would mind telling me about that ... commenting that medication often can make people feel tired in the way that she has described ... but then so too can depression ....*

Yes, I take a lot of medication, Mrs Pietroni, but I need it .... I was in hospital lots of times in Romania ... it was a terrible time .... The conditions there are primitive and for someone like me ... I am a sensitive person ... an intelligent person ... it was terrible ... truly terrible .... They do not have the treatment available in Romania that you have in England .... I know I am lucky to be here and to have Dr Thomas ... and the medication is better ... they don't have these things there ... but it makes me feel dreadful ... and I don't want to go back ... I don't ever want to go back ... those were terrible times ... I had dreams all the time .... I had hallucinations ... voices ... people speaking to me .... I felt terrible things were happening to me .... I ran around the streets shouting ... (*she laughs nervously*) .... I wanted to take my clothes off .... I was mad, Mrs Pietroni ... mad .... I don't want to be mad ever again .... I always take my medication ... I know I need it ... but I want a life ... it's not fair .... I know I am lucky but it's not fair that I should have to be like this when really I am an artist and I should be painting ... you know?

*As she speaks, she becomes more and more animated and I begin to feel engaged in her sense of outrage and dilemma, and her sense of unfairness, that someone with her vitality should have to be so devitalized in order to be kept sane. I can see what Dr Thomas had been driving at ... yet it seems a Catch 22 situation ... presumably if the medication were reduced Miriana would risk becoming ill again ... her current devitalized state is better than madness ... she seems quite clear about that .... At the end of her protest she slumps back into the chair and looks depressed again .... She is a refugee from her illness as well as from her country ....*

*I say I can understand why she is depressed because if she stops her medication her illness is likely to return, but if she carries on with it, she seems destined to sleep and feel tired all the time ... not much of a choice, is it?*

I have to do something ... I can't go on like this for the rest of my life .... I am still a young woman ... I would like to get married ... I would like to have children .... I must also return to my painting .... I like to see my friends ... I have some friends ... but usually I am too tired to see them ....

Sometimes at weekends I manage to go out a little ... you know .... I belong to a club for refugees and I meet people there ... it's a cultural club ... I am an intelligent person, Mrs Pietroni ... I like good conversation ... I like intelligent people ... I like Bohemian people .... I am an artist ... that is why the club is a good place for me to go to ....

*And so she goes on ... sometimes tailing off and looking at me to see if I have heard her message ... sometimes slumping into the chair .... It feels as if I am being shown the two sides of her ... the vital and the devitalized, the person who was hungry for life and the person who has almost been beaten by her inner experiences and what followed ... an experience from which she is now a refugee .... Time passed and I found myself feeling tired, very sad and somewhat impotent ... sure that I didn't yet know half of the story ... and yet also surprised at how much I had learnt from this first session .... Miriana had made her dilemma so clear ... and it was a felt dilemma .... She was emotionally present and as she said herself, she was intelligent. I began to feel irritated with Dr Thomas and myself because I knew the odds were strongly stacked against my being able to help, and yet now I felt I wanted to ... the Catch 22 had become mine .... I had no magic but I felt impelled to try ... more than that, I wanted to ... she had captivated me in some way ... she clearly had not given up on life or on people or ... more importantly, on herself ....*

*To Miriana I said, 'I recognize that so much of the life you would like to live has had to go on hold, because of your mental illness and the medication you need to keep the madness, as you call it, away. But you also convey very strongly that you have a life ... or at least part of a life ... and that you want very much to increase that part so that you can see more of your friends and perhaps begin to paint again ....'*

Yes ... but all I do is sleep .... I am always tired and when I am tired I can't paint ....

*At this point, I find myself feeling unsure ... is she really a painter? ....
Dr Thomas didn't mention it and she knows her well ... I've been captivated
by her ... perhaps I am being naïve? .... I say, 'You've mentioned your painting several times and it's clearly very important to you ... would you mind
telling me more about it?' Miriana explains that she's studied at a well-known
London art college and trained as a painter in Romania ... but on each
occasion she became ill and was unable to continue her studies ... but they
told her ... and she knew ... that she had talent .... I ask her what she
paints ....*

... she was motivated, verbal, had an
understandable problem ... so she met three of
our four selection criteria. But she was severely
mentally ill and I could only offer her six sessions
... what good could that possibly be and how
might I best use them? ....

My dreams *(giving a slightly
ambiguous laugh ... half embar-
rassment, half coquette)* .... I will
show you .... I haven't painted
for a long time now but I have
some photographs and I will
bring them to show you ....

*(Then more of the slumped-in-the-chair look.)*

*Thus I felt witness to the waxing and waning of her presence ... one minute
the person she could have been and then the person she is stuck with, knocked
out by medication and unable to think .... Yet through all this the message was
loud and clear ... she wants more ... she is motivated, verbal, had an understandable problem ... so she met three of our four selection criteria. But she
was severely mentally ill and I could only offer her six sessions ... what good
could that possibly be and how might I best use them? ....*

*I say I will see her again ... but it won't be possible for me to see her for
many sessions ... six at the most .... I will also want to speak with Dr Thomas
so that we could think together about her care .... Will Miriana give me permission to talk to the doctor about today's session?*

Mrs Pietroni, Dr Thomas explained that it was not possible to have
many sessions, but if you would see me just a few times perhaps it
would do some good ....

*'Well' I say, 'it might and it might not ... the problem is that your illness is
not going to go away as a result of seeing me and neither is it possible to give
up the medication and those are your two biggest problems ... as you have
described so clearly yourself ....'*

... just because I am mentally ill, Mrs Pietroni,
doesn't mean I don't have problems, if you know
what I mean ...

I know that is true .... I know
you can't do anything about that
... but I need to talk to someone
... just because I am mentally ill,
Mrs Pietroni, doesn't mean I
don't have problems, if you know what I mean ....

*I accept that ... I say ... 'I know, and can feel it's true ....*

*Perhaps what we should do is to meet not next week but in two weeks time,
after I've talked to Dr Thomas, and you've had some time to think about our*

*first meeting and what we could possibly do with just six sessions ... that's only five more ....'*

*As I say this, I realize I am committing myself to more than I'd intended ... but by now I feel more clinically sure .... I notice something unusual too ... GP, counsellor and patient for the moment share a common view with similar tensions about what is possible ....*

*We arrange to meet in two weeks time ... then I set up four six weekly sessions to stretch the time .... I draw this from the psychiatric outpatients clinic I witnessed many years ago in my psychiatric social work training.*

*This is the beginning of the Menu of Counselling Services .... After discussing the situation with my GP colleagues we decide to recognize the need for this type of intermittent counselling service in general practice which initially we call the 'psychiatric outpatient clinic' model ... later the Intermittent Service (D).*

## MIDDLE WORK

### The counsellor's story (Four years later: May 1997)

I am still seeing Miriana every six weeks ... we decided at the practice that a whole, new open-ended service was needed for patients with severe mental health problems ... and it has paid off ... her medication is much reduced, she's painting again ... and has had several exhibitions of her work and sold some paintings .... She also has several good relationships, including one with a man from her own country who seems to understand and care for her, and whom she brought to one session .... They argue about money ... about mental and physical space ... about clearing up the place and doing other household chores ... welcome, ordinary problems ... in contrast to the hallucinations of her past ....

I referred Miriana to the Community Mental Health team about eighteen months ago when I thought she could bear to state more publicly that she had a severe mental illness. The team provide her with group and individual support at a day centre, and regular review with a care manager and consultant psychiatrist. The diagnosis made by the consultant psychiatrist is manic-depressive illness or bi-polar affective disorder, but some doubt remains. The referring GP has left the practice and one of the other long-standing GPs has taken over. She and the practice nurse manage the still regular Modecate injections ....

Miriana has taught me and the practice a lot about counselling in general practice for people with severe mental health problems ... the experience of working with her made me revise the pattern of brief counselling which had been previously established ... I'll now see her as long as I work here ... and by using the intermittent service I've still seen her for relatively few sessions ....

... I learned from her that the essence of what general practice counselling can provide for people with mental illness is longterm, continued care of a limited but vital kind ... reliable continuity seems to be the key feature ....

I resisted pressure to close the case once Miriana had made a connection with the community mental health team, because I learned from her that the essence of what general practice counselling can provide for people with mental illness is long term, continued care of a limited but vital kind ... reliable continuity seems to be the key feature .... Life in the inner city for patients like Miriana would be more vulnerable without it ... there are fewer staff changes in general practice than in either social services or community mental health services ... we can almost guarantee continuity of counsellor, GP, practice nurse and receptionists ... over a long period of time ....

## The second GP's story (May 1997)

I don't know Miriana well but I have a sense of knowing her very well ... it's a bit of a contradiction I know, but let me explain .... I feel quite linked to her ... if I find she's on my list I'm interested ... I care about her ... it's as if I had a deeper or longer relationship with her .... I attribute that to what she invests in me ... she talks to me as if I'm the one she sees ... I'm important ... she gives very positive feedback about the help she receives although in reality I've done very little ... or so it seems to me .... I've probably only seen her a handful of times over the years but I was the one who first saw her when she registered .... When that happens I know I really focus ... I really listen in a different way to a new patient ... she may also have that connection with me ... but last year I probably saw her only twice .... I think the last one was when she came to see me for a housing letter ... I can't remember the exact circumstances without looking it up .... Oh yes ... I do remember now ... there was more to it than that ... she didn't turn up to view a place at the right time and then they were very punitive with her and said she would lose out and she felt they just weren't understanding that she has a mental health problem and sometimes can't wake up because of the medication and everything ....

I suppose one could say that she presents a reasonable story that arouses empathy ... she's very clear about her needs and very easily satisfied .... In fact she's very contained really ... she knows when she's had enough and is grateful for very little.

She has a psychiatrist, so I tend to be in the technician role ... prescribing or giving her depot injections ... she has her dose altered by the psychiatric team so I don't think I play a very active role in her mental health care .... She has a label now ... bipolar affective disorder

... but I really haven't seen swings ... she talks earnestly with me whether she's up or down ... even when she's down she's animated and articulate ... she tells you what she's feeling .... Because she's articulate, I wonder if I miss medical cues sometimes ... maybe I don't pick up things ... like that she's going down for example ... but then I think she tells her counsellor or the psychiatrist ....

Sometimes I give her her Depot injection and I think that's a very bonding thing ... it's very intimate ... I do it when the practice nurse is away or not available for some reason ....

Since 1995 she's got so much better ... there's no doubt in my mind that it's to do with the counselling ... she's had a predictable and regular contact over years now ... that's why it is ... but she's not really part of the community at all ... she lives separately ... I think of her engendering good feelings in all who see her ... but not really making contact ... I don't know really of course ....

I'm mostly talking about her positive projections ... which make her very attractive ... but there is something hollow ... not quite real ... yes ... hollow .... I see her walking down the street sometimes ... she always looks isolated to me ... very isolated .... She makes contact through her painting ... that's how she expresses herself ....

There was a study in Fulham on chronic mental health in the inner city ... where they worked out that a GP sees, on average, 11 patients like this a year ... the GP practices are where they're seen ... we're not really resourced for it, but we do it because we're interested and we have the skills here ... it makes it very rewarding ... but it is stressful ... very time consuming ... and we need to research it properly if we're to find out whether what we're doing is adequate ... there aren't any good pilot projects that I know of ....

As for the setting ... as well as the individual skills of the GPs and counsellors I think it's ... there's something about the support of the peer group we have here ... we have a kind of Balint-type group in our Wednesday lunchtime meetings .... I know he would turn in his grave if he knew what we do and yet still call it that ... and the purists would too, I know ... but we have a very cohesive and professional support group of physicians here ... that makes it possible for me to do my work ....

And as Miriana asks for so little ... even though theoretically it's less appropriate to her ... we do give her the time ... and my GP colleagues here have considerable experience of mental health problems which makes me feel I can carry things and take things on that I wouldn't otherwise .... I can't think of a diagnosis in which I wouldn't consider that

I had a part to play .... I hope I'm not arrogant but I'm not scared of taking difficult psychiatric problems on ....

Going back to Miriana for a moment ... there is a simple thing about her ... I think about her paintings quite a lot ... they're missives ... they're her contacts with the world ... I don't put them in her notes of course ... but it's not unusual to find a lovely card or even a framed painting sent with love ... I use them as bookmarks ... that's what I mean by her positive projections ... she shows how she's really alive when she paints ... but she's on the edge of everything ... she has to live her life in the city in a room ... struggling to exist in a non-psychiatric world ... she's so courageous ....

## The first receptionist's story (May 1997)

*This receptionist has been working for the practice for ten years, having joined the practice shortly after it opened in 1987.*

Miriana's very cheerful now ... always pleased to see us ... she always comments on how I look ... much more cheerful than she used to be .... She was very distant when she first came ... in a world of her own I would say ... her make-up used to be all over the place ... all smudged over her lips and her eyes ... she's quite a jolly person compared to what she used to be ....

When I first came she hardly used to say a word ... she seemed very sad ... then all of a sudden she came out of her shell ... perked up altogether ... and now she seems mostly happy to be here at the practice .... Mind you I often think that's a funny thing to be ... there's not many patients who'd be happy to be here, if you see what I mean .... I have no idea what's wrong with her ... she could have been a bit schizophrenic I suppose, but I don't know of course ....

As for how I think about her ... I always think it's nice to see her ... there's plenty out there make my heart drop when they walk in ... but I've always found her a nice person even when she's low ... she speaks very good English but I don't know where she comes from ... she never says a lot ... she's just pleased to be here ... as if she were visiting friends you could say ....

She did me a very nice painting at Christmas ... on glass ... very effective ... nice ... before she did what was like a child's painting and she used to keep asking me, 'Did you hang it up?' ... I didn't know what to say so I used to say ... 'Yes, of course' ... but now it's different ... I haven't seen her since Christmas ... I used to see her more often ... she never talks about the GP or her counselling to me ... though I always ask how she is and tell her how good she's looking ... which is true now ... to be honest I put it down to the counselling ... that's what it's all about, isn't it?

She doesn't see the GP very often at all now ... nor the practice nurse ... I don't know why .... She's not a weekly regular shall we say ... she sees the counsellor more regularly and as far as I know ... I don't think she's ever seen the complementary therapists ....

## A care planning review (CPR) in the community (May 1997)

*This review meeting is held some way from the health centre, and is attended exceptionally by the counsellor as part of the health centre's strong commitment to inter-agency collaboration, and to people like Miriana with long term mental health problems. The review is not held on the day the counsellor works at the health centre but it is possible to attend sometimes if informed of the dates. It takes about half an hour to cycle there from the university.*

### The consultant psychiatrist's story

So tell us how you are and what you want, Miriana .... Your contract here at the day centre has about another month to run ... then you can join the Leaver's Club which meets on a Sunday .... I'm not sure I can promise you the art group before then .... You need to finish what you're doing first .... We don't think it's a good thing for people to come here indefinitely .... They need to do some work and then move on ....

### The patient's story continued

Well, I am cross at having to wait for so long today .... I've been here since 2.15 and now it's nearly 4.30 ... why didn't anybody explain to me the time had been changed? .... I do have other things to do you know ... but I'm not ungrateful you know ... otherwise things are better .... I've been coming here as you know .... I would have liked to go to the art class because I am a trained artist and I don't really like doing these other things in the groups .... I don't mean to be offensive ... the people are all very nice but you know what I mean .... The other thing is I would like to see if I could cut down my medication a little more because I still feel too sleepy and I can't do my painting when I want to .... I am very grateful to everybody for what they do for me ....

### The consultant psychiatrist's story continued

We'll see if we can adjust your medication a little more ... but I don't want to take it down so far that you relapse ... it's pretty low already, but we'll have one more go at it .... I hear there have been a few problems with people here … one or two of the men … what was that all about? ….

Another thing … does anyone know what, if anything, has happened about Miriana's accommodation or the Home Office? Do we have the notes? …. Why don't we have the notes here? ….

… So … the plan is for Miriana to keep coming here and then to join the Leaver's Club in four weeks …. Next time I see you, Miriana … I'll review the medication again …. You'll take a bit more care with how you treat these young men here …. Giovanni, your care manager, will continue overseeing your care and the flexicare worker will continue … meanwhile you'll go on seeing Mrs Pietroni every six weeks or so and she'll come to the next review meeting … if it's on one of her university days perhaps she can bring the students … it would be good for them! Let's fix the date ….

## The counsellor's story continued

I was upset that Miriana hadn't been informed of the change of time arranged so that I could attend after my teaching at the university … it had been arranged some weeks before …. I wished I'd contacted her myself but at the time I didn't feel it was appropriate for me to liaise about the CPR meeting …. I was also stinging a bit about the only half-joking suggestion that I should bring my students to the meeting … all twenty of them? … many of them worked in mental health services anyway …. I felt the effort I had made to get there (and which I felt was right to make) had not been taken seriously …. I didn't feel treated as an equal ….

Going to the office of the community mental health team affected me in other ways too …. I'd recently undertaken some research which involved tracking nine mental health service users and their families and professional networks on three different acute provider sites over a six month period …. It had involved weeks of interviews and observational study …. I was surprised to see … when I entered the office … the white board on the wall for all to see … with the list of patients' names and their key nurses and psychiatrist … here … just like on the hospital wards … however Miriana was getting good drug supervision and was less alone ….

*The date of the next Care Planning Review Meeting, a few months later, is changed without letting the counsellor know, so she arrives on the original date and no-one is expecting her. The staff seem surprised that she's upset about this failure of communication and ask her to come the following week, but she is not able to. Miriana is soon after discharged from the day centre. The reviews continue with the community mental health team, but there are some changes of staff and communication is complex. Reports to and from the review meetings are exchanged and the community psychiatric nurse (CPN) continues in post and attends the practice Primary Care Team Meetings.*

## LATER WORK (SEPTEMBER 1997)

*One day, Miriana states in a counselling session that she has been offered regular psychotherapy by the psychotherapist on the community mental health team, and recognizes that this will mean an end to her six weekly counselling sessions, but it is what she has always wanted. This information had been flagged by a recent report from one of the CPR meetings ... so the practice counsellor is prepared and makes one further appointment in two weeks time to close. Counselling and psychotherapy cannot go on in parallel and she recognizes that this is a rare if unexpected opportunity for Miriana ... who however is disturbed by the change ... she doesn't keep her final appointment and doesn't respond to a nudge letter.*

*Soon after there are reports on the practice records that Miriana has been turning up at the Accident and Emergency department of a local hospital in the middle of the night ... very distressed .... Then all contact with her is lost for a few months. For the first time in four years, she stops coming in for her depot injections.*

## The first practice nurse's story (September 1997)

*This nurse has been at the practice for two and a half years.*

I can't quite remember the first time I saw Miriana ... I just remember that she has a very overt personality ... is very tall and quite concerned about her weight ... she always gets on the scales every time she comes in for her injection and she always comments on my weight too ... says 'you look great' or whatever .... She always has lots of energy .... I suppose that in two and a half years I've seen her about seven times when she comes in for her medication ... she used to come on a Friday before her counselling appointment but then my days off changed so she started seeing my colleague. We both do part-time ....

... you're not just there to give an injection are you? You have to be some sort of sounding board ....

She's someone you have to perform for ... I feel you have to put out that extra little bit for her because she's always so highly energized ... you have to psych yourself up because it always comes pouring out and you have to empathize ... you're not just there to give an injection are you? You have to be some sort of sounding board ....

We talked quite a bit if there was time ... she doesn't know I'm pregnant but we used to talk about getting older and getting pregnant ... I think she recognized that I was getting broody and had thought about what it would be like getting pregnant later in life herself ... then she had a miscarriage last year ... but she didn't want the baby ....

She was always very complimentary to me ... as with everybody .... I'm sure. It was sometimes like she had a love affair going on with me .... She always took lots of condoms away with her and we used to laugh about it but I don't think she felt safe with that man of hers ... and she was too insecure to have a baby herself .... She does stand out though, doesn't she? She was always talking about that accommodation of hers ... how unsuitable it was ... the cockroaches and everything ... I think it offended the artist in her ... she felt victimized by life in general I would say ... but she was always concerned about what she looked like and was very happy when she got that job in the Oxfam shop ... she used to sort the second-hand clothes. Then one day recently I went in there because I like second-hand clothes too and she wasn't there ... yet when I went in in the summer there were big kisses and lipstick everywhere ... I knew she was getting a bit hyper then ....

I was surprised to hear that she's come off her medication just recently because she always came in on time for it ... she knew she needed to come ... I wonder what happened?

The last time she came in for her treatment she was getting out of hand though .... She lifted me up in the air and held me there for a few seconds and I felt uncomfortable .... 'Anne, you're so lovely!' she said ... then she squeezed me by the hand very tight ... I thought she was getting a bit manic and I wondered if that environment that she lives in was tipping her over the edge .... I think that's what I thought ... I was uneasy ... you know?

But she seems intelligent and has a very good comprehension of what's the matter with her .... She's very articulate ... a very emotional soul I would say, a great feeler of things .... I couldn't say how much it's her personality and how much her illness that makes her that way .... Where are the demarcation lines anyway? Who's to say? On the whole, though, she was low because of the cockroaches and things like that ... she lives for her art and it was difficult in that room of hers ....

I felt that there was always that slight reluctance though ... or maybe it was sadness ... when she had to hop up on the couch and pull her pants down for the injection ... but she seemed to know it helps her a lot ....

## The second receptionist's story (November 1997)

*This receptionist has been at the practice for one year.*

Well ... Miriana is a tall, well-dressed lady with an air of discomfort about her face ... a nervousness somehow about her presence ... very

.... She needs a different approach if she's depressed or whatever .... I try to alleviate it .... I sense she's fragile and I know I've got to think ... to be cautious ... depending on the way she is ....

tense ... jittery .... I mainly talk to her on the phone ... and she always seems very grateful .... Then when I see her she's always very pleasant ... she makes me feel like I'm giving her a good service .... I'm aware of the way she is and always waiting to see how best to handle it ... because of her moods .... She needs a different approach if she's depressed or whatever .... I try to alleviate it .... I sense she's fragile and I know I've got to think ... to be cautious ... depending on the way she is .... I don't think she sees anyone except the counsellor and the doctor ... perhaps the nurse ... I'm not sure ....

I had a conversation with her yesterday, as it happened .... She was really motoring ... driven ... under pressure you could say .... She can be quite panicky when you talk with her ... there are a lot of problems under the surface ... I don't know what they are but I feel aware that she has problems .... At one stage, as I said, she was quite pleasant ... but recently ... very recently ... she's become more stressed again ... perhaps you could say she's a bit erratic in her behaviour ....

She doesn't worry about always seeing the same doctor ... she's more concerned with the length of time there is to wait ... there might be a problem with a prescription or a lower dose pill and she'll just settle to see the 'doctor' about it ... she rings up and really wants it there and then and I can't always do it .... One time she'd just seen the doctor, and she rang and was rambling ... hard to pin-point ... to be honest I had to wait and listen to try and find out what she wanted .... I don't know what her actual problem is, you see .... With most patients I don't know what their problem is ... just occasionally I know but there are so many ... it's usually okay to wait a couple of days ... but you have to be careful because her attitude can be one of just giving up ... that sort of attitude ... so we have to be careful ....

## The community psychiatric nurse's story (December 1997)

*This took place in an MHC primary health care team meeting.*

I can give you news of Miriana ... she's in the community psychiatric hospital .... I'm not quite sure how she got there but she's on the phone to her care manager every day and the consultant psychiatrist is looking after her .... She'd been going to A and E I think ... and doesn't want to go back into a bed-sitter but I think they're having difficulties finding anything else for her ... housing has completely dried up .... I hear it all because my desk faces her care manager's .... I'll see what's happened about her psychotherapy .... I know she did make a start but

I can give you news of Miriana … she's in the community psychiatric hospital …. I'm not quite sure how she got there ….
…. I don't know how you coped with her for all those years … she's very well known by everybody now ….

I'm not sure if she's still going …. I'll explain that you need to know … that it wouldn't be right to send her another counselling appointment if she's seeing him …. I'll find out …. I don't know how you coped with her for all those years … she's very well known by everybody now ….

## The second practice nurse's story (November 1997)

*This nurse has been in the practice for a year and a half.*

She's a refugee isn't she? …. Only last week I saw six or seven refugees … some of them are in a terrible way but others have a plan … one came and said he was going to 'disappear into Harlesden' … Look at poor old Kent Social Services … the NHS will crack too, you know, it will sink …. I used to work in the country and it's so different here in the inner city …. Just look at that meeting we've just had … real inner city stuff … so many refugees and services that don't connect properly with each other and people fall through the gaps ….

Last time I saw Miriana she was quite manic … having said that though … she's not always like that … the previous time was in June and she was quite childlike I would say … she wants care … she wants attention … she needs protection …. There was some man she said was using her and we talked about her walking away from him but she said she couldn't … she needed him too much …. 'I need the companionship,' she said, but she resented it too … he was an uneducated man, she said, worked with his hands and her own brother's a lawyer apparently so she's used to better things ….

She got pregnant last year around the time she was having terrible problems with this man … he disappeared for a while but kept coming back for occasional comfort and so on …. I tried to encourage her to find someone more suitable … she said he took her space from her … she always wanted to get her easel out and he didn't like it … she was planning an exhibition at the time …. I think she was also planning to go home … she had some royal connection or another with someone in exile or that's what she said and she was hoping to get them involved I think … she brought the photos of her work in for us to see … she has a real feeling for colour ….

She's a very tactile, touchy, kissy sort of person who needs a lot of approval, I would say … but she gives a lot too … compliments galore …. She's always welldressed although she gets her clothes second-hand … she has a good eye … but I think inside she feels quite the opposite … she comes in and says things like, 'That's a lovely scarf you're wearing' or 'I like the colour of your suit' and I think she wants the same kind of approval ... but she'll cry at the drop of a hat ... very emotional ... a typical artistic temperament in fact ... men, talent, temperament ... but I don't think she drinks .... I've seen her in cafés in dark glasses but I don't think she'd mix alcohol with her medication ... she's sensible enough not to do that ....

She usually comes in for her medication ... she'd stay and chat if I had time and sometimes I do have it but often I don't ... she's fine about her injections ... keen to keep them going ... knows she needs them .... I can't think what went wrong to prevent her coming recently .... It's so unlike her .... Around September/October there was an increase in the numbers of condoms she was getting from us ... but she has got standards ... I don't think it was anything like that ... I noticed her lipstick had started going beyond the edge of her lips ... perhaps she started feeling wild inside ....

If I had to say what sort of future I expected for her I'd have to say that I would expect her to go down ... I think she'll flounder in the end ... if we believe in research and everything ... I mean how is she going to keep her standards up? She needs a caring home ... she needs her art ... she wants to fulfil herself ... she's always saying that her family would be horrified if they saw how she's living ... she came from a good background, you know ... I suppose others are a priority and mental health goes to the bottom of the pile ... they all get lumped into what's available and it's not much anyway ....

Miriana is so different to that other patient I was talking about at the lunchtime meeting ... who was only seventeen ... also a refugee ... pregnant probably although she said it was the least of her worries. She told me, 'We will get a flat!' I gave her some condoms but her bloke virtually threw them back at me. But Miriana has no children, no family, lives in one room or used to until she was readmitted and for a while there were two of them in that room .... All she had was her art ... she's so different ....

## The patient's story continued (December 1997)

I'm so glad you could see me again Mrs Pietroni .... I've had a terrible time, a terrible time ... you wouldn't believe it ... I've been ill again ... they put me in hospital ... then they discharged me to some place at King's Cross for prostitutes ... it was frightening because of those men ... when Dr Jenson ... you remember my psychiatrist ... when she heard about it, she was very angry and they took me back into hospital a second time ... my medication is different ... but I've lost all my belongings can you believe it? ... my paintings ... all my paintings ... and I had an amber necklace that my parents sent me ... and although my clothes were second-hand ... they were good ... I chose them carefully ... for their colour ... now they are all gone because they wouldn't let me take them with me ... they were put in black plastic bags and into a social services store ... they said it was a long way away I think ... I don't know ... anyway when I was discharged they couldn't find them so I just have what I'm wearing .... Giovanni (*her care manager*) ... is trying to get me a grant but I think it is for bedclothes ... I know he doesn't believe I had all those things ... I had this friend who worked at Harrods and sometimes she used to get me things at the end of the sale ... she would put them on one side for me ... I know it's strange but I don't feel I can get better without them ... can you do anything? ....

*A week later*

There is a new problem .... I am in this hostel as you know ... it is out of the area ... am I going to have to go to another doctor, Mrs Pietroni? Will you be able to go on seeing me? I need you now ... I really need you ... I am frightened in the hostel because there are these refugees there whom we in my country consider to be very bad people ... a whole family, and cousins and everything ... last night this man was waiting for me on my doorstep and I was frightened ... thank goodness Giorg (*her former partner*) still comes to visit me once a week ... he's moved to Essex and it's not really allowed, you know ... but he has been very good to me and he says he will pay my telephone bill ... I made lots of overseas calls when I was ill ... I had to ... It's over two hundred pounds. I got into trouble for letting the bath overflow too ....

## The second GP's story continued

... No, of course we won't take Miriana off the list ... not unless she gets a permanent address somewhere out of the area but she's only in temporary accommodation now and likely to move back here somewhere if they can find her a place .... Yes, of course I'll write to social services about her belongings ... how terrible for her ... that's very serious ... we all know what her clothes meant to her, I think ....

## The counsellor's story continued

I arranged to see her every week until Christmas and then fortnightly after that .... The containment had broken down ... was it the natural rhythm of her illness ... or the discontinuity in her care and ending so suddenly with me? .... Or both? ... after her first few appointments with the psychotherapist she said she received a phone call to say she was unsuitable ... but I think they would have let me know ... she said she was struggling with the silences ... perhaps in retrospect I should have gone on seeing her every six weeks ... we shall never get to the bottom of it ... but we can help her get back on her feet again ... thank God for these sensible GPs ....

*Six months later*

*Miriana is in two year temporary accommodation with two rooms and has just recovered her belongings which someone found when they were clearing the store. Her medication is again being reduced. Her address is in our area, but she is to be transferred to another community mental health team because of the move. She is now coming to counselling sessions only once a month and is doing well ....*

## IN CONCLUSION ...

This story illustrates the following issues discussed in Parts 1 and 2:

### Containment

- The safety net of the practice team works for four years, then breaks down and is then recreated.
- The transformation achieved by the early work meets the patient's own goals of reduced medication, being able to paint again, and to have energy for friendships which are sustained even, to some extent, in her breakdown.
- The four- to six-weekly intermittent counselling service offers viable containment to a severely mentally ill woman.

### Multi-professional team

- Counselling is essential to the patient's changes, but is far from the sole contributor.
- Receptionists play a key role in containment and care.
- GPs and practice nurses give depot injections and offer thoughtful listening.
- CPN acts as link with the community mental health team.
- 'Inner team' is in the minds of each member in the practice, including the CPN.
- Primary health care team meetings play a vital part in communication.
- Problems occur between generalist and specialist agencies.

## Outcomes

- Medication is significantly reduced, meeting patient's and practice's needs.
- Patient's relationships develop and improve.
- Patient becomes able to work at her painting and to exhibit several times.

## Postmodernism

- Complexification: high numbers of staff and agencies each have different systems of belief and practice; individuals cannot know precisely what others are doing, or have an overview of how the patient uses different parts of the overall inter-agency system; lack of social services coterminosity with health services adds an important layer of complexity and instability in the care network, including changes of workers and offices.
- Global city: refugees in a London hostel for homeless persons are on different sides of a distant dispute.
- Commodification: costed community mental health care packages of limited duration are tied by service contracts charged to a fundholding general practice and monitored regularly; the cost of this patient's drugs is one factor in extending the counselling service on an intermittent basis to enable them to be reduced.
- Banalization: short term care contracts for mentally ill people deny the enduring nature of their problems and their need for long term reliable help in continuing relationships – 'people must move on'.
- Medieval inner city: the vulnerability of this isolated, mentally ill woman whose belongings are lost, who is then not believed, who is placed in a seedy hotel used as a King's Cross brothel, who is threatened by a male refugee on her own doorstep, who is periodically punished for aspects of her illness such as her sleeping patterns.

# 10

# Winter

*Alison Vaspe*

… Time, to make me grieve,
Part steals, lets part abide;
And shakes this fragile frame at eve
With throbbings of noontide.

Thomas Hardy, *I look into my glass*

---

## SYNOPSIS

This story begins in May 1994, when the counsellor has been
working at Marylebone for a month and is unfamiliar with the
general practice setting. She is completing the induction
programme for the counselling volunteer and supervision scheme,
which involves observation of GP surgeries and of reception (see
Chapter 3).

The patient is a woman of fifty seven. She lives alone and has
one grown-up son. She is seen for sixteen sessions in all, before
being taken on for psychotherapy on a reduced fee scheme. The
level of her depression and her fear of winter, both the reality of
long evenings and nights, and metaphorically, standing for old age
and the end stage of her life, lead the counsellor to manage the
available sessions carefully.

Four appointments hold the patient over the summer, and weekly
work (Service B) begins with the onset of autumn. The departure of
the patient's GP in November, together with her own decision to
pursue longer term psychotherapy, for which there is a waiting list,
make closing the counselling at this time inappropriate, particularly
with Christmas just around the corner. Instead, intermittent
sessions (Service D) hold the patient during the wait.

The patient's story tells of the loneliness and insecurity of city
life. The comfort of drink, drugs and sex mask the fragility of a
hand-to-mouth existence, a dependency on benefits and good will
for accommodation and support. The stories of the counsellor, two
GPs and the practice nurse who see her over these two years
convey the fragility of her defences, and reveal the tip of the
iceberg in a life of neglect and abuse.

## EARLY WORK

### The first GP's story (May 1994)

*Origins of the referral*

This woman worried me when she first came to the practice a few months ago .... She was angry with her former GP ... he seemed to have been quite tactless with her ... saying things about her age and how she didn't want to accept that she was getting on ... I remember looking at her and thinking, 'Well ... yes ... I can see that ... she is dressed younger than her age ... her hair is a bit too red ... a bit too dramatic against that pancake makeup .... But liking her too ... sympathizing with her .... Well ... who does want to just grow old? Why should she? I felt angry on her behalf ... and apart from that I thought her brave .... There's no denying her depression and loneliness ... no family to speak of and coming up to sixty .... She hasn't mentioned that to me ... not directly anyway ... but it must be around for her .... And she's not really responding to anti-depressants .... I wonder how she'd react if I suggested counselling ... I don't know .... Maybe I'll float the idea next time she comes in ... ask her if she wants to think about it and then come back if she wants me to go ahead with a referral ....

*The referral form*

Marjorie Holland. Born 22/2/37. Depressed. On sickness benefit: nervous debility. Worried about money and age. No previous psychological treatment.

Medication: Trimethoprin 200 mg but stopped after two doses as felt unwell on it.

Other Practitioners: none.

## The counsellor's story (June 1994)

*Receiving the referral*

I receive Marjorie's referral on a warm summer's day .... I know this GP ... Dr Han ... a quiet woman in her thirties ... calm and competent ... in contrast to the way I feel ... always rushed ... always in someone's way as I struggle to find notes or retrieve my appointments book from the cramped reception area ... always two steps behind at the GP meetings at which we discuss patients ... unsure which of the unfamiliar faces I see belong to new staff and which to people who have been around a long time but not on the days I'm in ....

I'll have to try to speak to her before meeting this patient .... I can't tell much from this form ....

## The records

First I look at Mrs Holland's notes to try to fill out the sparse information I've been given .... She's fairly new to the practice but has visited Dr Han a few times .... Depression from the first entry ... something about not liking what someone said about her age .... Lives alone ... one son under next of kin ... Church of England ....

I find myself forming an image of a widow ... perhaps an abandoned wife ... she might be dejected ... downtrodden ... the depression stemming from this ....

I'm trying to read between the lines but also to pretend these medical notes mean more to me than they do .... I want to get on top of the situation ... in fact I don't even know what some of the abbreviations mean ... can't even read some of the handwriting ....

What stays with me is the bare outline of depression ... being alone ... not liking what someone said to her about her age ....

## The first appointment (July 1994)

I'm in only one afternoon a week and don't manage to speak to Dr Han before the first session ... but as I go into my room to prepare to meet her I feel I should have made more effort ... I still feel very inhibited about talking to the other staff here ... still feel very new ....

I go to see if she's arrived .... There's a woman in the waiting area ... I ask for Mrs Holland and she stands up ....

I'm surprised ... disconcerted at her height .... She's not what I expect ... not at all the downtrodden figure of my expectations .... Large ... heavily built ... dressed fashionably in black trousers and a loose black shirt ... heavily made-up to look rather pale ... pallid .... There's something forbidding about her ... a suggestion that perhaps one should tread rather carefully .... Long wavy reddish hair ... untidy ... falling over her shoulders ....

Grey eyes meet mine without expression ... rather bloodshot .... She reaches out to shake my hand .... Hers feels cold in mine .... For an odd moment I think she looks like a man .... I introduce myself and ask her to follow me ....

## The patient's story (July 1994)

*She sits in the chair ... looks around ... seems composed ... folds her hands in her lap .... I ask if Dr Han has told her about the way we work at the Centre ... that we form a multi-professional team which means among other things that I'll be making brief notes following counselling sessions but that confidentiality is respected within the boundaries of the team as a whole .... Finally that I expect she knows there's a five pounds contribution towards the cost of counselling .... She interrupts me ....*

I ... I'm on benefit ... Do I have to pay?

*Her voice is rather high ... not like her appearance ... not confident ... but strained ... she sounds much younger than she looks ....*

*I say, 'No ... in that case of course not.' ... I realize I'm trying to soothe her ... feeling bad about talking about money ... perhaps Dr Han hadn't mentioned it .... I say more slowly, 'Dr Han has told me a little about you ... but perhaps you could start by telling me what brings you to counselling' ....*

*I listen as she starts to talk ... occasionally I nod or ask a question .... I'm conscious of a need to do this ... of a feeling of being flooded by her even though what she says is clear and quite coherent ....*

... Dr Han said I should tell you everything I can about myself ... you'll want to ask me a lot of questions ... I know that .... I have a son ... William ... he's illegitimate ... his father brought him up as part of his family but he ... William ... knows he's my son .... I told him when he was in his teens .... He didn't seem surprised ... he knew he had a different mother from his half-sisters ... maybe he even guessed .... Maybe I could have said something a bit earlier instead of waiting so long ... I don't know .... I don't know what he thinks about it ... we don't talk about things much .... But he wants to see me ... he's got a family of his own now ... maybe that's why .... He won't come to London ... to my place ... but he's keen on the children having a grandmother .... I don't know about that .... I'm not so good with children .... Not that they're not nice children ....

*Her voice still sounds strained .... It's difficult for her ... to talk about these very private things ... she's not used to talking about herself ....*

... I left home when I was seventeen .... These days I'd have been one of those kids around King's Cross .... I'd probably have gone on the game only I was lucky ... I found a job ... only told my parents where I was when I was settled and I knew they couldn't change my mind ....

It was Adrian who got me the job .... He's William's father .... He owned some shops ... fashion shops .... I was good-looking (*flatly, without emotion*) .... I looked good and I've always liked clothes ... I've an eye for fashion .... I worked for him and had a little flat over the shop .... It was fine ... fun ... for a while .... Only I got depressed when

I found I was pregnant .... I was paralysed ... I couldn't work ... just lay in bed .... So when William was born Adrian took him ... he said I could stay on in the shop if I wanted ....

I wasn't too sorry ... to be honest I was probably more relieved than anything .... It's only now I ... maybe if ... I don't know .... I'm not much good with children ....

*I say now ... with hindsight ... she regrets that it was too difficult to keep her son with her .... She looks at me and is close to tears .... She lifts her head ... then shakes it and goes on .... The sense of sadness remains ....*

I stopped working for Adrian .... The manager ... she helped me find something else .... I was doing other things too ... a bit of modelling ... consultancy ... that kind of thing .... I enjoyed that ... advising rich women what to wear mainly ... a bit of beauty therapy ... following the shows ... that kind of thing .... I really liked doing that kind of thing (*voice strained*) but now the firm's gone bankrupt ... three years ago ... and I got depressed again because I thought now I'm too old to start again ... who'd have me? (*No pause for breath, though she sounds on the verge of tears.*)

And I've still got my little flat .... Well it's Adrian's really but I'm a proper tenant and the rent's low .... He still visits of course ... we still have a relationship ... well ... he tells me about his problems ... his business ... his wife and children ... William ... why William doesn't want to see him ... what have I been saying about him ... and I don't .... Why should I? William makes his own decisions .... Why would he care what I think? (*She reaches for a tissue and blows her nose.*)

People seem to think I'm a tower of strength ... I don't know why .... I still look okay I suppose .... I look after myself and I dress well ... even if it is cast-offs .... My life's nothing to the things I hear from other women ... what they put up with! I've been lucky ... I look after myself ... I don't have to go along with things .... It's more what's ahead that gets me down .... That's what I said to Dr Han .... She's been very kind ....

*I think to myself. Time's going by .... She's told me a lot but it's hard to put it together in my mind .... So much to take in .... What's the central thing ... now? She's trying to tell me about how things are with her now .... Time's going by ....*

My doctor ... the other one ... not Dr Han ... she's been very kind ... my other doctor said I was denying it ... that I didn't want to know ... I didn't want to think I was coming up to sixty .... Well ... I said to him, 'No-one speaks to me like that' ....

*She acts the dialogue for me … her voice is cold and very angry …. I say again that time's going by and she's fearful about what lies ahead ….*

*She nods and says more calmly sometimes she doesn't know how she's going to get by … the picture seems very bleak … little in the way of savings … no prospect of work … one-way relationships that seem to offer little in the way of reliability ….*

*It's about halfway through the session …. I ask about her life before she came to London ….*

*She says nothing immediately … just sits looking at the crumpled tissue in her hand …. Then she speaks in a flat, emotionless voice ….*

*She tells me she's the elder of two children … she was born before the war and her brother Edward after …. Father was not much there when she was little … not very welcome when home on leave …. Mother was not interested … 'not much good with children' either … often out or taking the little girl on 'endless' visits to her own mother … the two women complaining about Marjorie's father while Marjorie sat quiet … dressed up 'like a little doll' …. Her mother, she said, had married beneath her … Marjorie had no idea why … just that her mother often spoke of what it had cost her …. But she doted on her son …. Both mother and grandmother doted on him …. By the time her father dies, aged fifty, Marjorie has left home …. Mother and grandmother 'ganged up' on her when she was about to leave school … wanted her to sign up for a secretarial course …. She knew she couldn't do that …. It just wasn't her ….*

*Towards the end of the session I return to the theme of what lies ahead and suggest counselling will give her time to begin to think about that …. There's a limit to what we can offer … up to about ten sessions … but we can make a start ….*

I've so little money I just barely get by …. My flat's lovely but it's always been damp and it gets so cold and now the ceiling's bulging and will probably have to come down …. Adrian's all right about getting it done but it'll mean workmen coming in and mess and noise but I have to do it or no-one will come to visit me any more (*again, the panicky tone*). Adrian will stop coming if there's a lot of mess. He hates mess …. It depresses him and I don't know what to do without the job … it's all I'm really good at … I can't stay on benefit for ever … but I'm too old … I don't think I can learn another skill …. I know I can't work in an office or like one of those women here … be a receptionist …. And when Mother asks me to go I can't say no any more … she's got no-one else now and she's not an easy person …. I don't know who else would stay with her …. I don't know what I'll do at her age … I can't see my son taking me in …. Well … he might … I don't think his wife would have it though ….

*I say time is running out and that we don't have much longer but that she's made a start …. She's frightened by the prospect of counselling … that it will be messy like the builders coming in … but she's come here to make a start at*

*looking at things … we can use the time we have left today to plan her coun-*
*selling sessions ….*

I don't know …. Yes … I would like to …. But I'm going to be away
… I said I'd visit my mother … then William …. (*Looks towards the pic-*
*ture on the wall which shows some geraniums.*) I love summer … it's my
favourite time of year …. I'm a summer person …. It's winter I dread
….

*I say, 'And it's your winter you want to talk about, isn't it?' …. I suggest a*
*second session for the following week … then two or three sessions over the*
*summer … then some weekly sessions …. I'm uncertain whether I'm doing*
*the right thing but recall my supervisor's comment on general practice … that*
*it has its own rhythm … 'flexibility with rigour' is her phrase ….*

*The patient takes out a powder compact and asks where the loo is …. Then*
*she thanks me and leaves ….*

## The counsellor's story continued

I have ten minutes before my next client …. I sit back and let my
impressions settle inside of me ….

I can still smell her perfume … a reminder of her powerful presence
…. I find the words 'a tower of strength' running through my mind …
yet in the session she seemed so helpless … overwhelmed … overwhelming …. She seemed to want to use this space though to talk
about how it feels to be a well-dressed doll … a cast-off ….

She's obviously frightened by her mother's condition and by what
lies in store for her …. We could look at this … it will be painful work
…. Will it be too much? Like the building work? No hope when she
spoke about that … more a sense of despair … counselling would be
like the builders coming in … mess and disruption … and for what?
She's told me she's a summer person ….

… I'm nearly out of time …. I need to clear my mind for my next
client …. But she lingers in my thoughts …. There's something else …
something she's not telling me …. Maybe to do with men … something
about 'going on the game' and modelling?

I put her file on the desk and prepare to look through my notes for
the next patient …. But I find myself still thinking of Marjorie Holland
…. I shouldn't have been so quick to say yes to the £5 not having to be
paid … it might seem like more under-the-counter clothes … cold charity …. Does she feel 'cast off' by Dr Han?

## The supervisor's story (July 1994)

This is a deeply unhappy woman … disturbed and terrified by the
approach of old age … after a lifetime of feeling left out in the cold …

turned into a doll by her mother ... and remaining one after the birth of her own child .... But she keeps herself out of things too ... with that chilling composure ....

Her 'tower of strength' is more like an iceberg ... her manner holds her together .... There's a kind of formality which hardens when she feels threatened ... becomes icy .... The lifeless tones in which she spoke of her childhood say something about how painful it is to look back on feelings that are frozen .... So the strength is precarious ... and there are likely to be other things going on ... feeling prostituted ... if not actually being so ... all only hinted at ... King's Cross, 'going on the game' ....

The question is how far she will be able to look at all of this? .... She may be a candidate for something longer term ... psychotherapy .... But how much can she afford? .... She seems motivated .... She might even be able to get herself into something ... with some help ... first the counsellor needs to see how the patient makes use of what's on offer here, though ....

I encourage the counsellor to talk to Dr Han .... There's a good relationship there ... it was a good referral ... the patient's trying to hang on to the 'good' here ....

There is a focus though ... facing her sixtieth birthday and the prospect of old age ... the winter of her life ... her mother and her facing an emotionally cold end to their lives ... trying meanwhile to keep up appearances ... two 'doll-women' .... She's confusing what's outside with what's missing inside ... and her comments about the builders coming in and the roof sagging are transference communications about her fear of what's opening up with the counsellor ... what it'll do to her relationship with Adrian ....

## The GP's story continued (July 1994)

Marjorie comes to see me a couple of days after her first counselling session ....

She needs some routine checks ... a smear test and a mammogram .... She looks as though she has something on her mind and I find myself wanting to ask her how it went .... I restrict myself to asking how she is ... as if to say I'm still interested .... I feel slightly awkward with her ... as though my role's changed ... but she looks pleased when I say that ... as though I've given her

Marjorie comes to see me a couple of days after her first counselling session ....
.... I find myself wanting to ask her how it went .... I restrict myself to asking how she is ... as if to say I'm still interested .... I feel slightly awkward with her ... as though my role's changed ... but she looks pleased when I say that ... as though I've given her permission to go on talking to me ....

permission to go on talking to me .... She's started swimming regularly ... she's very strict with herself she says ... goes first thing .... She's still worried about finding work but there's no way I think she's up to that just yet .... I suggest reducing the dose as a starter and extend her sickness benefit for another eight weeks ....

## The patient's story (July 1994)

*I do speak to Dr Han before the next session .... She tells me Marjorie has been to see her and seems pleased to be having counselling ....*

*This time Marjorie comes straight to my room and knocks .... Once inside she looks around and asks if it is damp ... it's almost cold in here ... I wonder if it feels like coming back to something ... from summer outside to thoughts of winter in here ....*

... I'm going to my mother next week ... I'm dreading it .... I suppose I always hope this time it'll be different ... that she'll be different with me but ... she'll just want me to run up and down for her .... Then she'll hit the bottle ....

*I say I wonder if Marjorie hadn't known if she was looking forward to coming here or dreading it either .... She carries on speaking but her eyes fill with tears and her voice is strained ....*

I did think about it .... I don't know ... I thought it might help to come before I went to my mother .... I thought about all I've said here .... I've talked about things I hadn't thought about for a long time .... That first session ... I was shaking afterwards .... But there are still things I haven't told you ....

Like my grandfather .... I always think of him when I go to my mother. I can't talk to her about it .... She'd just get angry ... but I can't just not think about it when it happened to *me* .... Because he ... he *abused* me when I was little ... and you keep reading about how abuse leaves lasting scars ... and I think that's true ... it has ... but if I talk about it to my mother she'll call me a liar or say I deserved it .... And he didn't do that much ... not like ... I've heard awful stories ... terrible things that have been done to people ... to children ....

*Her voice trails away .... I think carefully .... I don't want to say something bland and reassuring but it's more than that ... I don't want to break the thread of what she's saying .... It's as though she's put herself inside a capsule of memory and is speaking to me ... or herself ... from inside it ... and I'm the witness ... the one who listens and takes her seriously ....*

... I've only ever told one person about it ... one of my girlfriends ... we were drunk ... oh, years ago .... She told me she was abused by her father and I was shocked but then I heard myself say ... Oh ... you know ... and my grandfather abused me when I was nine .... And I don't know what I said after that but she never referred to it after that night .... I was probably too emotional ... it's usually me people confide in and when I do talk about myself it's too much ... I know it is ... I go over the top .... But you know it was such a shock the next day when I realized I'd let the cat out of the bag like that .... I hadn't even thought about it for so long .... I didn't know why I'd said it ... it's not as if I want to remember all that ....

*I say it's hard to tell me this and she's worried about whether she's doing the right thing.*

*She looks at me but I don't think she's really seeing me .... She goes on ... her voice is quiet but she's speaking now with feeling ....*

We went two or three times a year .... They only lived a few miles away but we'd always stay a few days .... Father didn't come of course ... my mother and grandmother would spend most of the time with my brother ... my grandfather would show me his things ... his medals and uniform ... things like that .... I loved it there .... It was a big house .... He let me drink little glasses of wine and port ... once he even let me suck one of his cigars .... And then his face would go red and he'd touch me ... put his hand on my arm and squeeze me or stroke my neck ... and his breathing would change and I'd stand very still ... so still ... it felt as though I had to or I'd break the spell ... and I never wanted to do that because I was his favourite .... Everyone knew that ... and that's why he did it .... It was our game .... And I know he loved me .... He never wanted to hurt me .... It was his game and I had my game and we knew that and we didn't ever spoil it ....

.... It was our game ....And I know he loved me .... He never wanted to hurt me .... It was his game and I had my game and we knew that and we didn't ever spoil it ....

(*Her eyes fill with tears.*) Only once my mother and my grandmother came in and I must have looked funny because they shouted at me and said I was bad through and through .... And after that I never went with them again .... I had to stay with my father and I didn't *like* that because he never liked me either .... I don't know ... I don't think he liked me .... If he did he never showed it ....

*Up until now it's felt as though it all happened yesterday ... the little doll playing her special game ... and then suddenly everything is shattered but she doesn't want to wake up ... it was better than what happened afterwards ... being sent to the despised father ... beyond the pale ... feeling nasty ... bad ... like coming to me? Sent by Dr Han when she wanted to talk to her some more?*

*I say carefully sometimes things feel wrong to a child but also nice ... but perhaps when her mother and grandmother said she was bad she believed it and believed she was no good or to blame? ....*

... There was only one other person who really liked me then ... a teacher at school .... She was the only teacher who did like me .... She was a bit of an ally really …. She was the domestic science teacher …. I was good at clothes then as well, I always liked sewing and things, and she encouraged me even though she was a bit old-fashioned you know … strict in that way …. I think she was a spinster … she lived with her sister …. She was kind but I don't think she was quite sure about me …. She wasn't used to teenagers really … I think … I think I shocked her a bit … made her feel uncomfortable ….

*I say maybe she's wondering if I'm shocked … whether I can understand how she must have felt? ….*

… Because I never expect people to understand me (*Her voice is high and tearful*) I don't know how to talk about myself …. Like when I went to the employment agency and I don't think they believed me … and I didn't want to say it was depression even though that's on the form … and all she said was I might have to retrain … so I suppose I'll have to learn computers and be in an office …. I'd like to work with people really but I don't know how …. I get too involved with their problems ….

*At the end of the session I return to the focus … of wondering what's in store for her as she grows older … and say we've set aside some time to think about that … but that today she's spoken of other parts of her life that are still very much alive for her … that she's carrying with her into the future …. I then confirm our next meeting ….*

*As she prepares to go Marjorie tells me about her session with Dr Han and asks if I will be talking to her about the counselling …. I confirm that we are in touch and she looks pleased ….*

## The counsellor's story continued (Summer 1994)

I'm a bit more optimistic after this session …. She's taking this time together seriously … trying to bring the strands of her life together … to find a way to speak of things she's wanted to bury …. Taking time for the unwanted part of her who's concentrated on the material things in life … just as she concentrated on her grandfather's big house and their special game so as not to feel just an unwanted little girl … or someone else's doll ….

Some kind of structure seems to be forming … there's less of that feeling of dread around … but I still feel uneasy ….

She comes for two more sessions in August and September …. These are less intense in nature as she reports on the few days spent with her son and then her mother …. She's touched by her son's efforts to accept her and treat her as one of the family but resentful at her mother's continuing demands on her … feeling she's treated like a servant ….

She's looking after herself physically … swimming … arranging for the building work on her flat to be carried out …. She comments poignantly that she can't imagine what it will feel like to have dry walls about her after thirty years of being cold and damp ....

These positive steps run parallel to a sense of foreboding ... the counselling room feels extra gloomy .... I find myself very aware of its lack of windows and the contrast with the summer streets above .... The subject of her grandfather is dropped and the present has taken over ....

Towards the end of September we start on the remaining weekly sessions we'd agreed earlier in the summer ....

## MIDDLE WORK

### The patient's story (Autumn 1994)

*Marjorie begins the first of the weekly sessions by talking about a visit to the benefits office which had left her feeling like a 'freak'.*

... Like my mother, she never understood me .... I couldn't have been a secretary. I'd suffocate in an office .... She never let me do what I wanted. I wanted to be a hairdresser but she wouldn't hear of it ... she was such a snob .... She just wanted me to marry .... She even had the man for me ... the son of our bank manager! Well ... I went out with him for a bit but I wouldn't have married him if you'd paid me ... not just him ... I couldn't see myself settling down and being someone's *wife* .... I was different ... I've always been different .... I'm a bit of a wild woman (*tossing her hair*) .... People look at me in the street but I don't mind .... I give them something to look at! I've still got my beautiful hair ... why should I pretend to be ordinary? If I've got nothing else I've got *style!*

*I say it sounds as though she never feels anyone is thinking of her feelings and feels quite wild about that ... so she tells herself she's special ... better that than feel outside of everything ....*

... (*Tearfully*) The only good thing that's happened to me all week is that I found this piece of material ... beautiful ... brocade ... almost as good as new .... I can make it up into a jacket ... it was just lying there ready to be thrown out and I took it .... I didn't care if they saw and thought, 'Oh, so she's reduced to that' .... So what? It was good cloth ....

I'll be seeing Adrian next week. I haven't seen him for two months ... he's been on holiday with his family and then he went on a business trip .... I might have it ready to wear by then .... *She gives a toss of her head and suddenly lifts her hand to her hair, catching up the long red coils and giving me a model's look ....*

### The counsellor's story continued

In supervision I realize I could have made a connection between

Marjorie's feeling that the only things she's entitled to are stolen pleasures ... cast-offs .... The stolen brocade .... Someone else's man ... and her yearning for maternal warmth and acceptance ....

The remainder of the session is largely taken up with Marjorie's relationship with her mother ... the lack of warmth and contact ... never remembering her mother putting her arms around her or saying she loved her ... her reliance on the bottle as a substitute for people .... I feel bogged down ... that the session is turning into a complaint .... That the focus is lost ....

This feeling also dominates the next two sessions .... I feel I'm offering coldness ... cold words rather than the comfort of the bottle or maternal warmth .... The relationship between us now seems saturated with her disappointment and despair ... the energy of the summer forgotten ....

## The patient's story continued

*When she comes for the fourth of the six weekly sessions she looks tired and frail ... for the first time I find myself faced with a woman who looks on the verge of being old ....*

*She is silent for a while after she sits down .... Then she tells me she has met someone she once had an affair with ... a younger man ....*

Well ... it wasn't that long ago ... last year in fact ... we had this fling .... He's a lot younger but the sex was good and we got on .... I always thought we could be happy together even though my friends told me I was crazy .... No-one approved of him .... They said he was a user ... and it's true ... he does take drugs ... hard drugs .... And I suppose ... I suppose to be honest I wasn't very happy at the time I was with him .... But on ... Saturday he was there and I ended up in bed with him ....

*She's speaking in the constrained voice of earlier sessions ... as though she wants to tell me this because it's important to talk about it .... This is in contrast to the complaining manner of the last two weeks .... Only as she says the last sentence does she give me a half-defiant look ....*

*I say she might think I disapprove too .... But maybe she also thinks I might be concerned by what she's telling me ... because here we are with just two more sessions to go and she's telling me how desperate she's feeling ....*

(*Tearful*) I was thinking about that ... what will I do? I was saying to myself, 'Who've I got?' There's William ... my mother I suppose .... But who cares about me? Who comes to my flat? At least Mark does ... he's very attentive when we're together ... and we enjoy ourselves ... we're good together ....

*She tells me more about Mark ... she thinks he's like a son for her ... that's why she finds him attractive .... But also he's weak ... a heroin addict .... He's thin and ill …. She knows he's dangerous … that he can't be trusted … however much she tries to tell herself otherwise ….*

*I say, 'And here I am … leaving you' ….*

*I return to the possibility of more counselling … somewhere else … if necessary take more sessions to think about it …. I explain that it would mean going to a counselling or psychotherapy agency which offered sessions at a reduced fee ….*

*She looks doubtful when I mention the fee and I remember my regret at not thinking about the £5 contribution for counselling when she started coming and wonder aloud how much she thinks she might be able to afford ….*

I don't know …. Really I exist on about £56 a week and there's nothing for me after bills …. I've just paid the gas … and I wrote to ask about their easy payment scheme because I find it easier to do it that way and there's not really anything for me (*tearful*) it's all a bit of a struggle … or I ask my brother for help with the heating in the winter … I don't know …. When Mark was going back on drugs last year I contacted a helpline thing and they sent me a list because I wasn't dealing with it very well … and the places charged anything from £60 down to about £15 … and I don't think I could afford anything like that … every week …. Maybe £5 … it'd be a struggle but I suppose I might manage that ….

*I say this sounds like something she wants to do … that there's a lot to come to terms with ….*

… Because I don't feel as bad as I did last year … this time last year … it's been hard … I haven't found it easy coming here (*tearful*) but I don't feel like I did then …. I mean … I felt good when Mark was there … good the other night … but in between … in between … when no-one's there … I just looked around me and I thought, 'I've got nothing … no-one' …. I didn't even feel upset … just cold and empty and thinking that … I've got no-one … only waiting for the next call … and my little nightly joint … but now … well … I seem to keep crying ….

*I say perhaps she might cut down on that nightly joint …. She looks at me for a long moment and I prepare to be given one of her icy put-downs … then she seems to take stock ….*

I suppose I could try …. To be honest … I've thought about that before …. Like when I'm watching a programme with families and thinking, 'Do I want to go on … sitting … smoking … waiting for the phone to ring … watching telly?' ….

*She ends the session with a return to thinking about the sexual abuse by her grandfather …. She always remembers it at Christmas, she says, but she also wonders why she should have to be the one to carry the burden and wonders how her brother would take it if she told him ….*

*When she goes I feel sad and worried about her …. I am also concerned that around this time the rhythms of general practice are making themselves felt with Dr Han's departure to have a baby .... Marjorie is attached to Dr Han and in view of this and the likelihood that a referral for psychotherapy will take time to come through I continue to offer counselling sessions on the intermittent pattern .... However, it also seems a good sign that she volunteered the information about her 'little nightly joint' ... with the implicit thought that perhaps the cost of that might go towards psychotherapy ....*

## LATER WORK

### The second GP's story (November 1994)

The first suggestion I should see Marjorie is in a meeting ... her name's familiar to me ... there's a sense she's been around for a time ... she's mostly seen Dr Han and she's being referred for psychotherapy ... the suggestion is that she could come to me for holding while waiting for that to come through.

It sounds a tricky situation ... trying to contain both these things ... the change of GP and the wait .... She's still having intermittent counselling sessions though ....

She turns out to be a large woman ... softly and carefully spoken ... but with an untamed look ... her hair is wild ... there's a lot of it ... she's dressed completely in black and I have a feeling ... as though there's this huge mass but it takes up so little space .... Afterwards I find a word for it ... like a black hole ....

---

**Figure 10.1**   The patient/GP/therapist triangle and associated transferences (from Jones et al 1994)

---

It is arguable that earlier writers were correct in placing the main emphasis on the therapist/patient relationship, and treating as irrelevant the Oedipal triangle formed by the patient/GP/therapist configuration [...] However, our contention is that these dynamics will be occurring in the patient/GP/therapist triangle and will be affecting the outcome of the work, whether the dynamics are consciously thought about or not; and the more these dynamics can be worked with, the more favourable the outcome is likely to be [...] In a general sense the patient referred for therapy in a GP practice is presented with at least a couple (therapist and GP), at most a group [...] The 'difficulties' of the team setting [provide] an opportunity to learn more about the patient [...]

[...] a referral begins with the transference to the GP which is in many cases powerful and positive. Sometimes referral to the therapist is only accepted by the patient because of the positive transference to the GP [...] Where the therapist works within the GP practice, the transferences remain linked and may be played out by the GP and the therapist. For the patient there is a development from a two-person to a three-person relationship with all that this implies unconsciously. In general terms, there is the potential to use this defensively by maintaining a split between the two, or to experience two parents working together harmoniously for his/her good [...]

She's not as demanding as I'd feared ... I'd expected there to be a lot to do .... She gives me the gratifying sense that I'm doing something important whilst actually not doing anything much ... and there is some actual physical doctoring to be done ... her leg was badly broken about thirty years ago ... it's flared up now with the cold weather we've been having ... she says her knee won't support her .... I spend a bit of time on the leg ... more than I usually would ... the physical touch seems to create a kind of contact between us that feels soothing for her .... I try strapping it but then I suggest she should see the osteopath ....

But her mood *is* very flat ... the tone of her voice ... it doesn't vary ... she seems resigned to this flatness ... resigned to her miserable state .... Everything comes across as very measured ... her depression comes across as measured too .... No floods of tears or anything ... nothing like that ....

Afterwards I just write very short entries in her notes .... I often write very full entries but I find myself not quite sure what I'm catching hold of ....

I have a sense of not wanting to sort of invade her ... just let her bring what she wants to bring .... Maybe that's another reason the notes are quite skimpy ... usually I'd have done a bit more digging .... I close the file thinking I should just let her bring what she brings ... let her feel okay about coming to see me ... just be there with her ....

> I have a sense of not wanting to sort of invade her ... just let her bring what she wants to bring ... I close the file thinking I should just let her bring what she brings ... let her feel okay about coming to see me ... just be there with her ....

## The osteopath's story (November 1994)

I'm not sure about this referral .... Dr Robinson said this lady wants some help for her leg ... when she comes in it's obvious she wants a disabled badge .... In fact I don't think the old injury's the problem at all .... It seems more muscular to me .... But I can see that's not what this lady's after .... I'll support her application for the badge ... it's obviously hurting her ... but I don't really think there's anything else I can do here or that she wants me to do ....

## LATER WORK
### The counsellor's story continued (to May 1995)

Marjorie finds the wait for an assessment for psychotherapy and the length of time between counselling sessions difficult .... In late November she's depressed enough to consider going back on anti-depressants …. I am able to offer her two appointments in December when she thinks about her Christmas plans …. Once again she feels the Cinderella of the family … she has to visit her mother while her brother goes on holiday abroad … then her son before returning to her empty flat ….

In the event she copes well and in January she's offered an assessment for psychotherapy …. That same month she decides to give up cannabis … but then, as luck would have it, her assessment is cancelled because of staff sickness ….

There are times during these months when I think she might give up hope altogether …. But she sticks to her resolution to give up smoking and is finally seen in May … by a man … in her letter she had requested a woman. However, she's offered psychotherapy and told they will be in touch to let her know when …. It could be a longish wait but by now she's made a good contact with Dr Robinson …. Her motivation is good …. There's no real need to carry on seeing her ….

Saying goodbye is hard … I want to ask her to let me know how she gets on … the theme of feeling cast off in favour of other patients comes up …. I acknowledge that the work has just started and that it's painful to say goodbye …. But the intermittent sessions also seem to have acted as a kind of weaning … there's some impatience and looking forward too … even though she still hasn't heard when she will be offered psychotherapy ….

## The receptionist's story (Autumn 1995)

I always found Marjorie very polite … but a bit … you know … haughty …. She's so striking … all that hair …. But as though it was saying 'look at me … but don't look at me' …. Not one of the ones you strike up a relationship with …. She must have been coming here over a year before I registered we were around the same age …. Funny … it suddenly occurred to me … I think it was because she looked sad …. Like she needed a friend …. And after that I began to notice her more … to say, 'Hallo, how are you?' She seemed to thaw out a bit …. Perhaps she just got used to me …. She stopped being so haughty …. She's always very polite though …. Not like some …. Some of them …. They come in …. 'I'm here to see Dr so-and-so' …. Like it's beneath them to have to tell you!

## The nurse's story (1996)

I saw Marjorie for a couple of times before I had any sense of depression …. It was after the counselling …. I do have a sense of when a patient's having counselling …. There's lots of writing in the notes and

I usually find I give them a little more time than usual .... But I think they keep it in their compartments ....

Usually the first time I see a patient I interview them ... after the questionnaire .... They never write anything worthwhile on it and some you don't really register ... others you can tell a mile off they've got problems!

This one has always presented as a very up together person ... it didn't occur to me that she might have problems ... Now she tells me about her aches and pains ....And this time we began to talk a bit more and I began to notice her more and be more open to her .... And that's gone on ....

This one has always presented as a very up together person ... she never said much and it didn't occur to me that she might have problems ....

Now she tells me about her aches and pains .... Then says, 'Oh well ... old age I suppose ...'

She was more open and I thought she looked very good for her age .... That she was keeping up appearances and doing *well*! And this time we began to talk a bit more and I began to notice her more and be more open to her .... And that's gone on .... She's just that much more talkative ....

## The second GP's story continued (1996)

What began to happen from about the spring and through the summer of 1995 is reflected by my notes ... there's a lot more written here ... they convey much more ... somewhere here I write, 'a definite feeling of empathy and therapeutic relationship developing' ....

I think there was some kind of watershed in our relationship ... my role for her started to feel more tangible ... she seemed more animated .... It was only afterwards that I realized this and made the link with the counselling coming to an end .... I don't really read the notes before seeing a patient who's having counselling ... I tend to read them afterwards .... I feel if I read them before there's a voyeuristic bit of me that wants to get involved in the counselling process and ask questions but then find myself having to say, 'No, no, you mustn't tell me this, you must tell your counsellor' .... But it's interesting that our relationship really did change when her counselling finished ... in May ....

And then of course she started psychotherapy in September .... I had some work to do dealing with her ambivalence in the first holiday break ... what's the point in going on ... that kind of thing ... and also again with her leg .... I found myself taking an unusually directive role over the summer break advising her to persevere and to keep going .... Because by that time I'd been seeing her for over a year .... I felt I had a sort of appropriate authority ... that she values my opinion ....

I find I'm beginning to enjoy seeing her and that she's revealing a bit more of herself to me ... although we don't talk about her issues .... There never feels any danger of that ... and after not seeing her for some months I put in the notes 'pleased to see her name on my list' ....

She looks different ... much neater ... her hair's done carefully ... so's her make-up .... She's still in black but a lot of people wear black and it doesn't seem as striking .... Probably because she's got more colour in her face ... there isn't that extraordinary contrast between her white face and black clothes ....

... I think one reason she's easy to see is that she doesn't demand anything ... there's a double edge to that because she's been very vulnerable and very depressed and at the same time she's been very much in control of herself .... I think she's probably always been quite contained with me .... I feel she's contributed a lot all the way through ... she's been prepared to bring her ... sort of quiet knowledge with her ... a sort of quiet wisdom about her ... a sort of sense that she hasn't been extinguished by her depression .... And now she's got a disability label which has helped her ... it's given her an added advantage in terms of her self-respect .... What she brings with her is ... I think ... that she's somehow maintained some sort of vestige of her self-respect ....

> I think ... that she's somehow maintained some sort of vestige of her self-respect ....
> Because if she'd been projecting the dependency into me I would have worried for me ... I'd have thought, 'Oh no, I'm going to be seeing a lot of her ... how am I going to manage her ....

I think in a way she's probably been very clear that I'm her GP .... That's why it hasn't been hard work or worrying .... Because if she'd been projecting the dependency into me I would have worried for me ... I'd have thought, 'Oh no, I'm going to be seeing a lot of her ... how's that going to be, how am I going to manage her?'

I've seen a transforming going on in her inner world ... not as a result of what went on between us ... it was the other way round ... changes in her internal world took place elsewhere and then our relationship changed .... So I was holding her while the transforming went on elsewhere ....

## IN CONCLUSION ...

This story illustrates the following issues discussed in Parts 1 and 2:

## Containment

- The flexible nature of the work holds the patient over the summer, before embarking on Service B when it is timely for her. Flexibility and sensitivity to the context are essential. Many problems arise when counsellors hold to a counsellor-centred view of the work, rather than a patient-centred view. A similar principle applied when counselling was extended following the GP's departure from the practice.
- Linking between the counsellor and the GP helped to prevent splitting (see Fig. 10.1).
- Referral to another agency entailed a longish wait. The combination of Service D intermittent sessions and a familiar GP provided containment of the safety net variety, following the transformative containing previously done by the counsellor. Many referrals for psychotherapy come unstuck because of the lack of a safety net, and because essential work on separation has not been done.
- The patient's relationships with the GP, the receptionist and the nurse provide continuity and ordinary contact alongside the new psychotherapy relationship. They give her space to come out of herself and respond to their interest and concern for her.

## Multi-professional team

- The counsellor's initial inhibition about speaking to the GP may have contributed to the patient's anxiety about being 'cast off'. The patient is visibly relieved when the link is made, at the end of the second session.
- The osteopath had doubts about the appropriateness of this referral, but held the boundary containing the patient by
  — supporting her application and acknowledging the real, if possibly psychosomatic, physical pain
  — keeping contact to a minimum and not wasting resources by offering more than the patient needs.

## Outcomes

- The GP and nurse have concerns about the patient, but are aware that her emotional needs are being taken care of in the counselling and psychotherapy. They are thus spared the full impact of her distress.
- Anti-depressant medication is reconsidered during the wait between in-house counselling and psychotherapy, but, with the

combined holding of her GP and ongoing Service D counselling sessions, the patient feels able to manage without it.

- The patient takes active steps to be responsible for her good health and to give up dangerous, unprotected sex and dependence on cannabis.

## Postmodernism

- Complexification/Medieval inner city: refugees from family distress who come to the city often end up homeless and/or 'on the game'.
- Medievalism: spurious identity and comfort are found through the illicit drugs market and its associated baronial sub-culture.
- Commodification of care: the referral is made to an independent charity, offering reduced fee psychotherapy, rather than to an NHS psychotherapy service. The patient is encouraged in her wish to take increased responsibility for her well-being, but difficulties include sustaining motivation, through cancellation of the assessment and delays caused by heavy use of a limited service, and potential splitting of the 'good object' of therapeutic work when going to an outside agency.

# 11

# The torture victim

*Alison Vaspe*

My reproach to some political discourses with which I am disillusioned is that they don't consider the individual as a value [...] That's why I say that, of course, political struggles for people that are exploited will continue, but they will continue maybe better if the main concern remains the individuality and particularity of the person.

Julia Kristeva In conversation with Rosalind Coward in *Desire*

---

## SYNOPSIS

This chapter tells the story of counselling offered to a political refugee, who is suffering a living nightmare in which he is in fear of his life. Through his contacts with a sympathetic but firm GP, who suggests counselling as an alternative to anti-depressants, he gains the courage to talk about being tortured and imprisoned and, as painful in a different way, being exiled from his country. When the patient does not return following the first fifty minute session, which is clearly too long and painful for him to bear, the thirty minute sessions of Service E, some three months later, provide some space for the memories behind his nightmares to come to the surface. Containment is first of the safety net variety, and then is transformational.

---

## EARLY WORK

### The nurse's story (December 1995)

I gave Ibrahim his health check when he joined us .... He told me he was from Sudan and was a political refugee .... I asked about where he was living and all that and he told me ... but really he didn't say much about himself .... Just that he had family in London and he doesn't like where he's living .... And that he wanted to find work .... I remember the way he said that ... he was so determined to get something but I felt a bit depressed about it because his English wasn't very good .... That might have been because he was depressed though ... he looked it ... depressed and somehow haunted .... I really felt for him .... I just checked his blood pressure and all that ... weight ... diet ... he was dia-

.... I think he was mainly depressed and told him I thought he needed to see the doctor about that .... He said he would but no-one knew him when I mentioned him at the Process Meeting .... It was a couple of months before I saw him again .... I saw that Dr Shah had taken him on .... She was seeing him quite often and I felt relieved ....

betic and didn't look well ... but he seemed to be eating all right .... I think he was mainly depressed and I told him I thought he needed to see the doctor about that .... He said he would but no-one knew him when I mentioned him at the Process Meeting .... It was a couple of months before I saw him again .... He needed a blood test and I saw that Dr Shah had taken him on .... She was seeing him quite often and I felt relieved ....

## The GP's story (September 1996)

### Origins of the referral

I remember when he first came in ... nearly a year ago ... it was just all these medical problems. Diet ... he was diabetic ... we had all that stuff investigated. Then after three or four consultations he started opening up ....

I can't remember exactly what the first thing was ... I don't think he came out with it straight ... but it was some stress-related symptom that emerged ... it hadn't emerged before ... not how horrific it was ... and I know I felt irritated ... hassled ... so much to deal with on the medical side and now all this comes out .... But that's my problem, I know, not his ....

As I get to know him ... I don't know how often he's been in ... several times ... sometimes he forgets or oversleeps ... but I'm warming to him ... feeling empathy for this guy who I thought had such a calm character when I first met him. And the relationship's improving as time goes on ... on two levels .... We're always dealing with two levels ... the medical stuff as well as all this ....

What he told me was awful .... I wanted to refer him to a clinic for post-traumatic stress disorder ... to deal with it ... because I didn't think the counsellors would be able to offer him enough sessions ... but having spoken to Liz (Dr Robinson, the senior partner) about it ... we just don't have the funding ....

Because counselling ... someone being seen *here* ... can give you a kind of heartsink feeling ... an extra load I suppose ... it's challenging .... But he needs something ... he needs time to talk about it ... about the nightmares ....

Because counselling ... someone being seen *here* ... can give you a kind of heartsink feeling ... an extra load I suppose ... it's challenging .... But he needs something ... he needs time to talk about it ... about the nightmares ....

*The referral form*

Ibrahim Kader. Age 37. Depressed following imprisonment and torture. Refugee from North Africa. In this country 4 years. Political asylum. Suffering from nightmares and stress. Headaches.

Medication: Fluoxetine 20 mg (started August).

Other practitioners involved: no, but housing problems / social services.

## The receptionist's story (October 1996)

I remember Ibrahim came in and said he had an appointment to see the counsellor .... He didn't look too happy about it. I made sure he sat in the right place and said the counsellor would be with him soon .... I always take care of him when he comes in ... he's a lost soul isn't he? .... I look out for him and make sure he knows where he's going ....

... he had an appointment to see the counsellor
... I made sure he sat in the right place ...
.... I always take care of him when he comes in
... he's a lost soul isn't he? ....
I look out for him and make sure he knows
where he's going ....

## The counsellor's story (October 1996)

I receive the blue patient request form ten days after Dr Shah completed her referral .... The waiting list is mounting but I have a space coming up in two weeks .... I take the referral from the file ... see the name and wonder ... must be Muslim ... where's he from? Then I read 'political refugee' and think of the newspaper I was reading yesterday morning ... sitting in the bus ... a picture of a church in France and the word in the headline ... asylum .... This is news for us too ... the rules are being tightened ... no wonder this man is worried ....

I will be able to see him at least three times before Christmas .... Then I'll be away for a week .... Will three sessions be enough to hold him through the break? It'll need addressing well in advance ....

*Discussing the referral*

I send the appointment letter and catch Dr Shah in reception ... tell her I will see Ibrahim in two weeks time .... She looks worried when I mention him and says she hopes he'll come .... He needs to talk to someone but sometimes forgets appointments .... I ask about his status as a refugee but she says that's fine ... no worries there ... only the housing's a problem and he wants to move ... his flatmate's the problem ....

She has a patient to see and hurries off .... I am left with uncertainty .... I didn't ask about the torture .... I don't know how damaged this man will be ... perhaps he won't come .... Then I realize I am half hoping this patient won't come .... This needs thinking about ... this resistance ... my fear ....

Torture ... I have a jumble of thoughts about what that could mean .... I think of fingernails being pulled out ... beatings ... brutalities on the body ... pain .... I go to the notes and see he was beaten and in solitary confinement .... I think of a woman trade unionist I worked with some years ago when I was in publishing ... she was in solitary confinement for six months ... and still traumatized all those years later ... still suffered from spells of amnesia .... This man was in jail for forty days, six weeks .... But he was beaten .... I try but can't think what that was like ... I can't imagine ... the fear ... the pain ....

## The patient's story (November 1996)

*I see a youngish Arab man as I take some notes through ... standing a little hunched by the wall ... I know it's him somehow, but check with reception anyway ....*

*I go up to him and introduce myself .... I say his name and ask whether I'm saying it properly and he nods ....*

*I explain where the room is and lead the way .... As I wait by the door I see he's limping ... not very much but with a slight dip in his walk and a feeling of dragging himself .... I show him the chair and he looks around him at the walls before sitting down and looking at me ....*

*He looks Arab ... black but not very black ... A word comes to mind ... impassive ... stoical ... but at the same time it's obvious he's in pain .... I don't yet know whether it can be talked about ....*

I am here because Dr Shah says I should talk ....

*I speak slowly and clearly .... I say I've spoken to Dr Shah .... That I'd like to hear his own story .... My words seem to stay close to me ... I have a sense of not being heard ... which is uncomfortable .... I'm wondering if he's understood me when he begins to tell me his story ....*

I have ... nightmares .... Someone chasing me ... a man ... he has a gun ... a knife ... there is no escape ... only to fall ... I am in a high building ... the only escape is to fall into the sea ....

*His voice is slow and there is no life as he speaks .... I say he's having terrifying dreams .... As though he can't escape from his memories ....*

And I have headaches ... I do not sleep .... It is very bad ....

*I ask him to tell me his story .... Slowly and with difficulty he tells me ... that his family is in Sudan ... his mother and sisters .... He is not the youngest ... but the next to youngest .... He was a student ... he left home to study in France ... foreign affairs ... his first time away from home .... His father is dead ... he died when Ibrahim was four ... maybe five .... Ibrahim had a fiancée who married someone else after he was freed from prison ... he was in prison in Sudan for forty days for being in the student union in France ... he was alone in prison ... he was beaten ....*

Now I cannot return ... my family ... they get me out and I am here four years .... I am political asylum .... No ... I have no worry about the law .... I am political refugee .... I have flat but it is not ... good ... my flatmate ... we have arguments ....

It is just ... who will clean up ... we do not agree ....

*He looks a little shamefaced and smiles .... For a moment I see the younger brother in him ....*

I want home of my own ... family ... children ... work .... I apply for work in public administration .... I have not succeeded yet ....

I am worried about ... my health .... I do not sleep .... I am ... irritated when I talk to my sister .... She is here ... yes ... in London .... I see her and her family ... her husband ... yes, I can talk to him ... but I do not speak to him about ... what is ... here ....

*He hits his hand against his heart ....*

I am irritated with her when I speak on the phone ... because I do not sleep ... I have nightmares .... I dream of people who want to kill me ....

I do not talk ... I do not tell people what is in my heart ....

Dr Shah says I should talk about it ....

The pills did not help .... No .... Dr Shah says I should talk about it ....

*The session is long and full of silences .... I feel futile ... my questions and responses pointless ... as though I'm causing him further suffering by keeping him here .... By the end I have a bare outline of his family situation and of the reasons for his nightmares .... But I haven't been able to respond to the need he's brought to me ....*

*I wonder whether it's difficult for him to talk to a white woman .... Dr Shah is Asian .... What does that mean to him, I wonder? ....*

*In answer he says no ... it's not that .... Again he says he doesn't talk much to people about what's in his heart .... After another long silence he says Dr Shah wants to stop his pills .... I say I'll be talking to her and will tell her he's mentioned the pills ... but that he can also see her and ask her about this .... He says the pills didn't help and again that Dr Shah had said he should talk about it .... I say this is a place to talk with me about these things ... this nightmare from which he can't escape .... I offer him two appointments for the two following weeks ....*

## The counsellor's story continued (December 1996)

Ibrahim doesn't come for the sessions we booked for December and makes no contact with the practice .... I write to him offering another date but I don't hear from him .... I speak to Dr Shah about the missed appointments, stressing that I'll see him again if and when he wants to .... It's a time of year when referrals are piling up so I leave it at that ....

## The GP's story continued (January 1997)

Ibrahim comes in asking about anti-depressants ... he doesn't say anything about the counselling .... I know he hasn't been attending .... I make out a new prescription for Prozac .... When I ask about the counselling he says he doesn't find it easy to talk about things .... I ask if it's the language ... he says it's not .... I try to push him on with it although he says he doesn't want to talk .... I feel I'm trying to hold on to something myself but ... that it will all come together ... in the end .... I hope it will .... I'll keep pushing him on ....

Then I tell him I'm going to be leaving the practice ... I hope for a little while only ... I don't know .... He seems a little sad because we do have a relationship ... he does seem sad that I'm going ....

I'm left with ... all the medical side of it ... that's never quite got sorted out ... someone will have to push on with it .... He needs that ... he's not like some patients ... some of them don't need any help to get what they need ... but he does ....

## The counsellor's story continued (February 1997)

Dr Shah tells me Ibrahim wants to book another appointment with me ... she thinks he will be able to talk now .... I have a half-hour session available and offer him this .... I explain in the letter that it will be for thirty minutes ... that this is all I have but that I can offer it now .... Thinking back to the session we had, I also think thirty minutes might be a better time for him ... more bearable ....

## The patient's story continued (February 1997)

*He does come for this appointment .... I say it's been some time ... November ... but I understand from Dr Shah that he wants to talk now .... He looks at me and again I can't make out if he's understood what I've said ....*

No ... I do not *like* to talk ... but I know I must try ....

*Silence .... He looks away ... just the clock quietly ticking .... He sits with his legs crossed ... hunched forward a little ... he sits so still ... and I sit still also .... I wait ... concentrating on finding some mental space to hear him in .... It's very difficult to wait for him to speak ... not to know what he'll tell me ....*

*After a long time I say it's difficult to find the words ....*

*He jumps when I speak ... then looks shaken ... as though jolted awake ....*

No ... it is all right .... It is difficult ... but I want to talk ... to *you* ....

*He looks at me .... He's helping me out .... Suddenly I realize that of course it's not the words that are the difficulty ... it's the gap between his feelings ... his tortured state of mind ... and my inexperience of such things ... such unimaginable things ....*

*Now I can hold his gaze ... the feeling is very intense and I can only think I must hold on to it ....*

*He's looking around him ... at the narrow room and barrel-shaped ceiling .... Suddenly he looks haunted ... fearful .... He looks around at the walls ... the ceiling ... he becomes agitated and suddenly twists his head as though he fears someone will come up behind him ....*

*It's as though he's in another place ... somewhere I can't follow ... except I also feel he's saying this to me ... with his movements ... like a mime ... he's showing me something ....*

*I say it's as if we're in his nightmares ... the nightmares he described to me ....*

Yes ... the nightmares .... Yes ... I dream they are coming to kill me .... I sleep little ... I have headaches ....

... the nightmares ....
... I dream they are coming to kill me ... I sleep little ... I have headaches ....
It's difficult ... but I will try ... I want to talk to you ....
Just me and you ....

*He starts to look around again ... at the walls ... the ceiling ... turns his head to look behind him ....*

*I look at the white walls ... the narrow white walls and barrel-shaped ceiling of the crypt .... I say the room's small ... there are no windows .... I wonder if it seems like a prison ....*

Yes ... the prison .... It is like that ....

*He looks sharply around him again then turns suddenly to stare at me before crying out:*

I don't know why they want to kill me ....

*I feel a shock of fear and then a feeling of unreality ... again the air is thick around me .... I can't think ... yet I feel I must put the sound of my voice in the room .... I say, 'It's impossible to understand why anyone wants to kill you' .... The words sound meaningless ... stupid and inadequate .... Still, I say again, 'It's impossible to understand ... but we can make time for you to try to speak about it' .... He looks at the clock behind him and I say, 'Today we have to stop .... It's difficult to speak about this nightmare ... not only the language' ....*

**Figure 11.1**   Shared experience and language (from Stern 1985)

Many experiences of self-with-other fall into [an] unverbalized category: mutually gazing into another's eyes without speaking qualifies [...] But [...] with language, infants for the first time can share their personal experience of the world with others, including 'being with' others in intimacy, isolation, loneliness, fear, awe, and love...

It is difficult … but I will try …. I want to talk to you ….
*He points at me.*
Just me and you ….
*I offer him another appointment …. He says he'll try …. It's early but he'll try to get up …. He can't sleep at night and then he can't get up …. I say I'll offer him a later time if one comes up …. He says okay … then he rises and limps slowly away ….*

## MIDDLE WORK

### The supervisor's story (February 1997)

In supervision the counsellor speaks intensely of her experience of being with Ibrahim in that vaulted room with bars on the windows … of how she feels he's taken over by memories … the nightmare … of being in prison … in fear of his life ….

I take some time to consider with her the importance … not only of the torture and the fear … but also of the massive loss he's experienced … the loss of his role … his life … mother … fiancée … his whole sense of safety ….

He has put into the counsellor … very powerfully … the unimaginable nightmare he's been through …. She's been taken over by torture and it's been difficult to speak and to think …. But we need to understand more about what he's lost …. He's a young man … a son … fatherless … an only son … a student … perhaps a firebrand … perhaps not … we don't know …. But the counsellor needs to feel able to ask … to get to know the real person he is and was … to be interested in him in an ordinary way … like with any other patient … to press him on the

**Figure 11.2** The alienation of torture victims (from Summerfield 1996)

[. .] many of the survivors of torture do not start from a standpoint which we can easily identify as individually psychological […] They start from the standpoint of their horror and their perplexity about the destruction of their social world. That does not mean that in their own terms they do not have a psychological view. The question is about their psychological norms rooted in their cultural background and how they touch ours. This is an exquisite thing, a power problem. We would hate to put our words into their mouths at the very time when they may be speechless about what's been done to their worlds. And we would seem the opposite of what they had been, we are intact, we are in power, we are salaried, we are whole […] They have lost their world, they are statistics, they are a marginal person in Britain […] They have lost touch with a culture in the year within which they knew who they were […] And to [the] extent they can rebuild a social world, each citizen will draw from it his or her resilience, their psychologcal capacity […] Their capacity to problem solving and activity and aspiration […]

facts about his life … the close practical detail … to find out more about the then-world and try to make the connections with now ….

I say she needs to get hold of the part of him that feels distraught … to imagine a baby who's been sent away … to hospital … to be prodded and poked … investigated and operated on … hurt …. A baby who's terrified … who needs to find out how to be safe on the knee again …. She can be quite firm … sympathetic but firm … for example … why can't he get up in the morning to come for a counselling session? …. It's a lifeline ….

She looks shocked … she tells me she feels two things … a kind of shocked outrage … that it is … almost taboo … to think of him like this … as a young man with problems that she might try to soothe as a mother would her baby …. She says … intensely … *'He's a torture victim … he needs special treatment ….'* I say first he's a human being … next he's a torture victim …. *'You need to hold the memory of the whole human being to help him feel whole again ….'* I see the counsellor begin to relax a little ….

She begins to think about him … to feel curious about him as a young man … the life he led … what he wanted from it and why he did what he did … she comes up with a couple of things he'd said that she'd forgotten … about his father dying and about not speaking of things that were close to his heart …. About his fiancée marrying someone else … while he was in prison being tortured ….

## The counsellor's story continued (March 1997)

Ibrahim doesn't turn up for his next appointment but phones later in the morning to say he's sorry … he had a sleepless night … he would like to come again …. I say I can see him next week at the same time ….

## The patient's story continued (March 1997)

*When he arrives he apologizes for not coming the previous week ….*

I have nightmares …. I do not sleep ….

*He falls silent and looks around him … at the walls … at the clock behind him ….*

I do not sleep … I talk to my friends … not … about this …. I stay with them to not go … back … I stay with them until late ….

*I feel his deep sadness … a young man … out but not enjoying himself … afraid to go home … without a home to go to. I say he stays with his friends … not to talk but so as not to go back to the nightmare … but here he comes to talk … to talk about the nightmare ….*

I do not want to talk … but I know I must ….

*His face is blank … and I feel blank … cold ….*

I was ... taken ... for my ... activity ... I was in a room ... a small room ... I was ... alone ....

*The word fades in the air .... I say, 'You were alone .... No-one to talk to ... or to defend you' ....*

I was held there ... it was very alone .... But they ... beat me .... My back ... my legs .... For long ... then ... release ... my family ... they get me out ... they get me ... here ....

*He looks at me .... I feel oddly visible ... too white again ... strange ... as if I were in the glow of a light .... He speaks passionately ....*

I hate it here .... When I came ... I was lost ... people ... hurrying ....

*I say, 'White people ... hurrying white people ... white ... like me' ....*

I was lost ... only my sister ... my mother ... cannot come ....

*I say he was without the important people in his life ... in a new life that was strange ... surrounded by strangers ... like me ....*

I want family ... home .... My fiancée .... She came ... she is married ... she is here ... in London ... she was here ... before ... I wait to become ... for political asylum ... she did not wait for me ....

*It's a while before I can take in this extra blow ... that she not only didn't wait for him but was in London ... with someone else .... I say slowly, 'She married someone else ... and she's here with him ... you had that loss as well' ....*

I wait .... I live ... only to be there ... to return .... I wait ... I listen ... for change of government .... Like before ....

*He is looking at me ... suddenly I see him differently .... I know little about the affairs of his country .... But this is a man with a cause ... a different man from the broken person I have also seen ....*

*I say he hates being here ... talking about the loss of his mother ... his country ... his fiancée who didn't wait for him to come out of prison ... but now he's chosen to ... been driven to ... by loneliness and fear .... We have to stop but next week ... and for some weeks after that ... he can come and take his time to go on talking ....*

*He nods ... stands up ... leaves the room .... Then he holds out his hand and looks at me .... I shake his hand and he goes ....*

## LATER WORK

### The counsellor's story continued (Spring 1997)

Ibrahim comes nearly every week after this session ... for nine sessions in all .... The theme continues ... fear ... and loss ... but also he speaks more of his yearning for his mother and his home ....

The nightmares continue ... the same ones he came with ... about being chased and in fear of his life ....

He says he mixes with other exiles and talks with them about the political situation but not of what is in his heart ....

A plan takes shape to see his mother ... not in the UK as she can't come here ... but in a neutral country ... at present she's still in Sudan ....

He misses a couple of sessions and then doesn't come for two weeks running .... I write to him saying I'll hold one more session open for him .... He comes the following week ....

## The patient's story continued (June 1997)

*He tells me he's moved out of the area into a new flat .... Now he's closer to his sister and friends but he knows he'll have to register with a new GP .... He hopes to find a counsellor there ....*

*He speaks with feeling about the plan to see his mother in the summer and ends by talking of the health centre ....*

This beautiful place ....

*He mentions Dr Shah, who is still away .... He wants to come back and visit ... to thank Dr Shah for talking to him ... he does not talk easily to people and it has been important. The counselling has been important .... He pauses ....*

This has been important .... To talk here ....

*He looks around the room and for a moment he is lost again ... the fear returns ... he looks behind him and I say, 'The counselling has been important but there have been terrible memories ... the room has been like returning to the prison cell.' ....*

*He steadies himself and looks at me ....*

No ... I see now ... I see it is different .... It is not so like that room ....

*We speak about his future .... He knows of the Medical Foundation for Victims of Torture and says if he can't find a GP with a counsellor he will go there to talk more .... I offer to help if he runs into problems over finding someone ....*

*It's time to end .... I say this .... I feel awkward ... uncomfortable .... I see tears in his eyes .... I have tears too .... I feel I should find a better way to speak about the experience he's had ... of this place ... of London ... that it's been hateful as well as important ... but I can't ... not now ....*

*We shake hands when he goes and there is warmth in the formality .... I feel a sense of having lost something which stays with me through the day .... I won't know how his story ends ... but he's moving to better accommodation and has his own plans for the future .... That's London ... people move on ....*

.... I won't know how his story ends ... but he's moving to better accommodation and has his own plans for the future .... That's London ... people move on ....

## IN CONCLUSION ...

This story illustrates the following issues discussed in Parts 1 and 2:

## Containment

- The safety net of nurse, GP and receptionist holds the patient within the practice at different points of need.
- The GP contains the patient's need to talk, despite his fear of doing so, when the counselling link is too fragile and difficult the first time.
- The supervisor helps the counsellor to grasp the whole person with all his losses, and not just the torture victim, and to contain the patient's mixed feelings about talking.
- Transformation does occur by the end of ten sessions. The patient can see both the room and the counsellor differently, and is more in charge of his life.

## Multi-professional team

- The process meeting provides the opportunity for the nurse to express her concern about the patient to the team as a whole, and to alert the multi-professional team to his needs.
- The GP builds a relationship with the patient until she thinks he is ready to talk in counselling.
- Ongoing communication between GP and counsellor helps keep counselling open as an option for the patient, in spite of the difficulties.

## Outcomes

- Medication fails to help the patient's problems with sleeping and headaches.
- Counselling provides an alternative to medication.
- The nightmares continue, but the patient begins to reconnect with his passionate desires to be active on behalf of his country, and to see his mother again.
- The patient's feelings of someone and something good resurface through the counselling relationship, and give him strength to move on.

## Postmodernism

- Global city: refugees are housed together but cannot always talk about traumas they may have experienced.
- Medieval inner city: people are herded together as refugees and may be excluded from the broader community.
- Banalization: awarding the patient a stereotypical victim status inhibits the counsellor from thinking about him as an individual.

- Complexification: housing provision is limited, and the offer of improved accommodation takes priority over the advantages of remaining in a general practice in which the patient has begun to feel well contained by a network of different team members.

# 12

# The uprooted schoolgirl

*Alison Vaspe*

[...]one word, one phrase is enough, one of those ancient phrases heard and repeated an infinite number of times [...] for us to pick up in a moment our old intimacy and our childhood [...] These phrases are our Latin, the vocabulary of our days gone by, our Egyptian hieroglyphics or Babylonian symbols. They are the evidence of a vital nucleus which has ceased to exist, but which survives in its texts salvaged from the fury of the waters and the corrosion of time [...]

Natalia Ginzburg, *Family sayings*

## SYNOPSIS

This chapter is about a seventeen-year-old girl making the transition between school and college. The referral for counselling was made following a panic attack which prevented her from attending a college entrance interview. The Menu of Counselling Services was by now more firmly in place, and the counsellor offered ten weekly sessions (Service B) with holiday breaks around the midpoint; a further interruption came about as a result of the counsellor falling ill. The work shows the importance of arranging all sessions in advance, especially where transitions are a key issue. As a result, despite interruptions, planned and unplanned, the patient had a sense of the ten sessions acting as a dependable bridge that would carry her from one point to another. The form of containment is transformative, with the patient becoming more able to bring together words and feelings, past experience and present reality.

## EARLY WORK
### The GP's story (April 1997)

This is the first time Athena's been to see me on her own ... she's a sort of petite ... rather frightened ... slightly elfin-like little waif .... Very different from her parents ... her mother ... she's very confident ... a little agitated ... but very confident ... and her father ... a steady man ...

moves at a different pace from the mother ... very calm ... very steady ... he spends a lot of time in Greece ....

She's very anxious ... there's a prospect of some sort of interview ... she doesn't want to go .... I can see immediately this is going to need some more in-depth work .... There's exam anxiety mixed in there somewhere too ... she seems quite paralysed by it all ... quite seriously affected by it .... I suggest counselling .... I'm not sure if she'll take it up ... when she goes I find myself thinking about her parents more than her ... she doesn't take up much space ....

.... I can see immediately this is going to need some more in-depth work ....
There's exam anxiety mixed in there somewhere too ... she seems ... quite seriously affected .... I suggest counselling ... I'm not sure if she'll take it up ...
... she doesn't take up much space ....

### The referral form

Athena Kouros. Age 17. Low mood following panic attack. Only child of parents with high expectations. Starting college October. Wants to chat. No other practitioners involved. No previous psychological help. No psychiatric history.

## The counsellor's story (April 1997)

The referral is made at a time when the counselling team is operating a waiting list of up to six weeks .... Athena will be sitting her A levels by the time I have some sessions to offer .... Before sending her a 'wait letter' I therefore have a word with Dr Robinson who says she will be seeing Athena the following week .... She offers to discuss the delay with her and to see her on a holding basis until her exams are over .... I think this is a good solution .... Offering counselling before the exams would either have to be work focused or would be likely to affect her concentration .... In May I send Athena an appointment for mid-June ....

I receive no confirmation of the appointment but the preparation Dr Robinson has been doing with Athena and also her young age decide me to keep the session free .... I tell reception I'll be in the counsellors' office and that I'm expecting Athena .... I then attend to some paper work .... After a couple of minutes I'm called to the phone .... Athena is calling to tell me that her mother has reminded her she's supposed to have her appointment this morning ... she's on her way in ....

When I go to collect Athena I find a neat, thin, anxious-looking girl holding a handbag on her lap .... She smiles politely when I introduce myself .... In the counselling room she sits where I show her ... still holding her handbag .... She keeps it on her knee as I tell her about the counselling arrangements .... I draw out what I'm saying a little as I want to give her a chance to settle into the session .... Then I say Dr Robinson has told me a little but that I'd really like to hear from her what brings her for counselling ....

## The patient's story (June 1997)

(*Hesitantly*) I had an interview ... for college .... I panicked .... But I'm all right now .... I've been accepted at another place and I'm going there in the autumn ....

*Her voice has a slight accent ... not really Greek ... more north London ... but very careful ... an odd mixture of the streetwise and the demure .... It's rather painful to hear her voice ... her mouth is dry ....*

*I say the referral was quite a long time ago and that she's had quite a wait for this appointment .... She tells me it doesn't matter and that she's over it now, but the silence following this quickly becomes uncomfortable .... I have to make a conscious effort not to speak into the silence but to remain open to anything more she might have to say ....*

> .... I don't know if you can help me ....
> ... I'm all right now ... I'm pleased with the college I'm going to instead .... I just don't want it to happen again ....

(*Awkwardly*) I had to give a talk ... and I couldn't do it ... I knew I couldn't do it ... I couldn't get up in front of people like that .... I didn't know what to do ... I just knew I couldn't do it ....

I told my mother in the end .... I didn't go to the interview ....

*She falls silent but seems to be thinking what to say next ....*

I ... I'm just a bit worried it'll happen again .... I don't know if you can help me .... I mean, I'm all right now ... I'm pleased with the college I'm going to instead .... I just don't want it to happen again ....

*I say it sounds as though it might help to talk more about what happened and ask if she can tell me about it in a bit more detail .... I start her off by recapping what she's told me ... she got an interview to her first choice of college and then she was told she'd have to give a talk ....*

I didn't know what to do when I saw that ... I ... I just didn't know what to do .... I felt ill when I thought about it .... I thought I must be crazy. I didn't know what was the matter with me .... I ... I got to the point of taking a bottle of vodka to school with me ... not a big bottle ... I just drank a bit before class ....

*I ask if she's done that before ... if she drinks much ... and she tells me she doesn't drink regularly ... she hasn't got a good head for drink .... She just did it because she'd read a story in a magazine once about someone keeping a bottle of spirits in her bag to give her Dutch courage .... She'd been frightened by the way she was feeling .... She couldn't understand it .... She'd never liked read-*

*ing in class but it had never been as bad as this .... It was her mother who sug-gested going to the doctor .... She hadn't expected anyone to suggest coun-selling ....*

*I comment on this ... saying she'd even forgotten her session .... She gives a small smile and then looks serious and worried again ....*

I was a bit worried .... But I know I need to do something about myself ....

*When I ask about her family background she blushes slightly and says in a rush that she's more like her father ... she gets on with him better ... her moth-er's the confident one while he's quieter .... Her mother makes her angry because she compares Athena to the successful ones ... the exam successes .... She pauses ... then says that it was her mother she talked to about the inter-view ... though ....*

*She describes her mother and father .... Her mother's a maths teacher in a boys' school and her father is Greek .... Athena is an only child ... her mother had two miscarriages before her ... and carried on working after having her .... A nanny looked after her as a baby ... she was Greek and Athena spoke no English until she came to London ....*

... My mother spoke Greek to my father and me .... I didn't speak English at all until we came to London and I went to a school ... a rough school .... I learned English there .... I forgot nearly all my Greek .... I only speak it now with my father .... But mostly we speak English now ....

*The word 'rough' lodges in my mind .... I find myself thinking of a school of hard knocks ... perhaps Athena's experience ... roughly knocked off balance ... by change and disruption ... to her language too ... her father's language ....*

*I ask about the nanny and Athena tells me she was left behind .... I com-ment on the further loss and disruption and she looks sad for a moment .... But she remains half-poised on the edge of her seat ... leaning a little to one side ... still holding her handbag ... as though on the edge of something but unsure which way to go ....*

*I say it must seem odd talking about it ... all these years later ... maybe painful ....*

*She responds by saying she doesn't usually talk about things .... She doesn't really have many friends and gets on better with boys than girls .... 'But I'm not really close to anyone' ....*

*I say it was her mother she talked to about the interview and maybe it's difficult to talk to someone else .... She looks at me and says in a rush that sometimes she can talk to her mother but she's not really close to her ....*

She's so critical of me .... She criticizes my clothes ... my hair ... *(imi-tating her)* 'Why are you wearing that colour? ... Why do you tie your hair back that way?' .... *(Pause.)* She's only happy when I'm successful ....

*I say maybe she thinks I'll be critical and she says slowly she does find it hard to talk to people …. She always feels there's something wrong with her when she starts talking about herself …. Then she leans forward and takes something from her bag ….*

I … I think I have a social phobia …. I read about it …. It sounded like what I've got from the way they described it ….

*She unfolds a piece of paper …. It looks like a photocopy from a magazine …. As I reach out to take it I feel the pathos of this self-diagnosis … the scrap of paper with its worn creases … the neat handbag … the loneliness she is describing ….*

*I hold the piece of paper … it's from a woman's magazine … not one of the teen magazines but written for another generation … her mother's generation ….*

*Holding the paper open on my lap I acknowledge the difficulty of coming here and talking about these things when perhaps she'd hoped that her doctor would give her a cure … make the feelings go away …. Then I suggest that she comes again and that we book in some sessions … and that we'll need to think about the period between leaving school and starting college in October ….*

## The supervisor's story (July 1997)

In supervision the counsellor discusses a schoolgirl she's seen a couple of times …. A girl with a very extreme form of performance anxiety … she gives a brief account of the two sessions … it seems to be difficult to speak about her … some inhibition … her presentation is uncharacteristically stiff ….

My first, unhelpful thought is that this would be a classic case for brief focal therapy … thirty sessions … David Malan-style … if she had any money that is ….

There's a focal problem … an understandable history … a psychologically minded patient who is engaging with the counselling … an interesting young woman …. Sometimes I wish it were possible to do weekly work for this period of time … but resources don't permit it ….

…. It's crucial to avoid replicating the loss of the nanny … although … the patient may do this herself and cut the counselling off prematurely ….

However, the patient is very fearful and her need now is to be held safely and firmly for as long as possible …. It's crucial to avoid replicating the loss of her nanny … or rather to work with it clearly … although of course the patient may do this herself and cut the counselling off prematurely …. I suggest fixing times with her and even saying at the beginning that there's going to be a replication of the pattern … that she'll lose her counsellor at the start of a new life just as she lost her nanny when she came to London …. But also examining what she makes of this ….

There's a lot of significant history here ... but we don't really know too much about what the nanny was like ....

Then the switch between countries is so sudden ... the miscarriages are also important ... maybe there were stillbirths ... they might have fed into the mother's harshness ... failed mourning ... hence a need for Athena to be successful ... even a boy .... And what about the Greek connection ... the father? ....

The choice of the design course is also interesting ... she would have known a different alphabet ... as though there's something residual that wants to be worked on at the interface between art and language ... trying to find a language that can bring the parts of her together? As though there's a bridge that needs to be made? ... at present she's logged into another culture ... her father's ... in the child part of her ....

The public pressure came when she was just not ready ... her reaction was harsh but also healthy ... she's not yet found her language ....

## MIDDLE WORK

### The counsellor's story (July 1997)

Over the four weekly sessions before my holiday break Athena begins to tell me about her difficulties with friends at school .... She seems to have divided them up into two groups .... One made up of girls she feels are better off than her family and who she's envious of ... the other of girls who are more rough and ready .... That word again, 'rough'.

This division of friends seems related to her rather distant mother of childhood ... relatively rarely seen and seeming out of Athena and her nanny's league ... and her 'rough and ready' nanny .... This pattern seems to be repeated in the process of choosing her college ... her first choice a centre of excellence which she could not aspire to ... and the college she'll go to in October ... still good but less prestigious ... more ordinary-sounding ... more accepting of her perhaps ....

I begin to take on board just how devastating the uprooting must have been for Athena ... and at the same time I begin to find myself a little less tongue-tied with her ... less lost for words ....

---

**Figure 12.1** Replication of past experience (from Freud 1914, pp. 158–159)

[...] the patient *remembers* nothing of what is forgotten and repressed, but [...] he [sic] expresses it in *action*. He reproduces it not in his memory but in his behaviour; he repeats it, without of course knowing that he is repeating it [...] at last one understands that it is his way of remembering [...]

I say Athena's still caught in that gap between her childhood nanny and a mother who wants to bring her up as a little English girl .... However I find it hard to gain a sense of what her father wants .... A man whose first language is Athena's first language .... In my mind's eye I have an image of the three of them sitting round a table talking in English ... awkwardly ... like three adults .... This is encapsulated by Athena talking about her mother's reasons for the strict English-only regime ....

*She said it was to make up for lost time ... that I should have learned English sooner ... it's my mother tongue ....*

I feel intense sadness when I hear this and also sense her confusion .... I say that English is her mother's tongue ... but it's not the language of her childhood .... She says no ... but she's not a child now .... Now English is her language .... And we sit in silence ... caught in the fracture of two languages ... two periods of time .... I find myself wondering if she'll return after the break and realize I haven't found out if Dr Robinson will be here when I'm away .... I've got absorbed in the dynamic of abandonment ....

I say she probably feels I'm abandoning her .... She tells me she lies awake in the night debating whether to come for her counselling session and that a part of her says it's better to be a hermit than go through 'all this' ... better to have nothing than risk being rejected ....

I say she thinks it would be better to reject counselling by not coming and that way someone else will feel abandoned ... me .... She nods ....

*Athena cancels her next session in a letter saying she's decided to go abroad with some friends from school and telling me when she'll be back .... I write confirming her next appointment ....*

## LATER WORK

### The GP's story (August 1997)

Athena's mother tells me she's done well in her exams .... She seemed surprised .... I felt a bit surprised too ... and pleased ... that she got as far as counselling .... I wasn't sure she'd get very far with it ... or be able to use it ... she seemed so timid .... From her mother's account she seems to have moved very quickly ....

### The patient's story (August 1997)

*She arrives fifteen minutes late ... looking confident and tanned ... her brown hair streaked with blonde ... she's wearing a stylish outfit ... a little black suit .... When she sits down she hesitates and smiles ... then shakes her head ....*

I don't know what to say now ... after such a long time ... three weeks .... One thing I can say is ... I'm feeling all right now ... really .... I suppose it was being on holiday ... having lots to do and think about ... distractions ....

*She looks confident but her voice is tight ... the familiar difficulty in speaking .... I feel anxious ... rather cold in this room ... unwanted now perhaps ....*

I suppose the only thing that's worrying me is ... I've been worrying I might lose the friends I've made recently ... from school ... and ... I'm a bit worried about college ....

*I say perhaps she doesn't want to lose the past ... the friends who've been important to her ... but it's hard to hang onto it ... easier to leave it behind and pretend she's not bothered ... like telling me it's only three weeks since the last session when in fact it's over a month ... and arriving quarter of an hour late ... as though unsure whether to renew this old acquaintance ... belonging to two worlds is difficult ....*

I did wonder .... It was all right when it was every week but after ... a month ... I suppose I didn't want to talk about things I haven't been thinking about .... I didn't want to remember I wasn't normal ... that I have problems .... I was thinking about when I went to my new school and I didn't make any friends .... I didn't like anyone .... I kept thinking ... will I do the same thing at art college? Even my friends from school ... I don't know how to stay in touch .... I want them to be the ones who ring me ... I don't want to phone them first ... but I suppose if they're real friends we'll stay in touch .... I suppose we've got things in common ....

*She asks how many sessions we have left and we take a moment to book them in .... Then she talks about her parents ....*

I'm not really talking to them about things now .... Like ... I'm not really thinking about what it'll be like when my father goes to Greece ... I mean .... I'm thinking about it and I know I'll feel sad ... but ... I feel sad but I don't feel sad .... It's odd ... I know I should feel sad but I don't .... Although I did dream about it a little while ago .... It was upsetting ... that we weren't all living together any more ....

*I didn't know her father was leaving London ... for a moment I feel dismay ... shock ... why didn't I guess some kind of separation between her parents was on the cards? But then I pull myself together .... I realize that despite not wanting to know she has decided to come and talk about it .... It's pretty fundamental ....*

*The rest of the session is spent talking about her father leaving ... Athena's guilt, sadness ... anger ... and her mixed feelings about being left alone with her mother; the two of them alone together ... almost for the first time ever ....*

*In some ways she says she can't see what difference it'll make ... that she's always thought her parents rather cold with each other ... more like friends than anything else .... But they never talked about separating ... they never talked about it together as a family ... about how they felt ... how she felt ....*

## The patient's story (Autumn 1997)

*Athena comes for two more sessions .... In the first she says she wants to put all her feelings behind her ....*

I just want to get on with my life ... but I'm still worried .... What if something like that happens again ... if I can't ... fit in ... at college? ....

*She seems caught between two worlds again .... I say it seems impossible to think she might find a place there to talk to someone ... about her feelings ... like she has here ... about fitting in ... in new surroundings ....*

.... she's talking to her mother more now ... ... talking about things makes a difference .... .... she's glad to have a safety net here at the health centre ...

*She tells me at least she's talking to her mother more now ... also that she's seen there's a counselling service at college ... she thinks counselling helps her to handle things better ... talking about things makes a difference ....*

*She cancels her next session by letter as she's in Greece with her father .... She confirms her next appointment but unfortunately I have to cancel this important session because of illness ....*

## The receptionist's story (October 1997)

I think Athena's notes have gone .... She's moved hasn't she? I don't remember her really ... she was that quiet girl .... I remember her parents ... her father especially ... he's quiet too I suppose .... I don't really remember her though ....

---

**Figure 12.2**  Development and change in young people (from Noonan 1983, pp. 5–6)

Personal maturation requires some things to be yielded to make way for new ones; it requires us to convert childhood into a memory which is alive, if not palpable, inside us, and this means we have to mourn aspects of our child-self so they may be internalized. Change and gain involve the same ambivalent process as loss does: space needs to be made for new experience, just as the gap created by loss needs to be bridged. In both, continuity is established by looking back longingly to how it was, and looking ahead uncertainly to life as it will be, and continually reinterpreting ourselves and the world in the light of new developments. Not to do so, not to spend time and energy on weaving this individual thread of meaning, leaves us in a falsely based, defensive existence, where the whole aim becomes simply to survive change [...]

## The patient's story (Winter 1997)

*I write on my return confirming the next booked session the following week and sending good wishes for her first week at college .... She doesn't come but four weeks later leaves a message asking me to ring her at home ... can she come for a session during Reading Week? ....*

*She tells me she's settling in well at college and making friends ....*

I wonder ... maybe it's too good to last ... will it all go wrong for me? ....

*Her relationship with her mother continues to improve but Athena sometimes feels as though she's acting a part .... She says she's glad to have a safety net here at the health centre ... we make another follow-up appointment for a little before Christmas ....*

*Athena does not attend this session but sends me a letter after the event ....*

I'm doing fine here. I still think I might go to the counselling service for students here ....

*I feel after all I have been shown what it feels like to be abandoned ... but she's also telling me she's all right and is able to find a place to talk about things if she needs to again ....*

## IN CONCLUSION ...

This story illustrates the following issues discussed in Parts 1 and 2:

### Containment

- The GP contains the patient when the counsellor is unable to send an appointment.
- Beginning counselling when the patient is sitting exams would have been impractical.
- The supervisor provides words to contain the patient's wordless communication of how it feels to be uprooted and unable to communicate.
- The counsellor contains the patient's inner division well enough for her to manage the transition and to achieve a viable transformation.

### Multi-professional team

- The GP uses counselling skills to support the patient through her exams, and prepares the ground for counselling.
- The patient impacts very little on other members of the multi-professional team, although other family members are seen.

## Outcomes

- Talking to the GP helps the patient avoid alternative ways of coping, such as use of or dependence on alcohol.
- The patient repeats her own experience of being abandoned, and avoids coming for a closing session in which to say goodbye, but she takes forward the knowledge that she can express herself in words and be listened to, and her feelings respected and understood.

## Postmodernism

- Global city: this young woman is caught between cultures and languages, and continuously repeats the split between old and new.
- Commodification: she feels she has to package and sell herself as an adult for the college interview and in the sessions, with her grown-up handbag and magazine article, but feels a confused and frightened child inside.
- Banalization: the break-up of her parents is treated by the family as if it were a footnote, mentioned only in passing, as if it were unimportant. Perhaps the loss of her nanny was treated similarly.
- Crisis in authority and leadership/loss of generational differences: a young girl is treated like an adult, as if she must manage this difficult transition in her life (and its precursors) like her mother's clone, denying the pain and confusion and the uncertainty of adolescence.

# 13

# The fractured widow

*Marilyn Pietroni*

Had we grown old together, I might have slid more gently into age; You would have altered: toughed by autumn's frost To a more sober russet.

Margaret Hamilton Noël-Paton, War widow in *Chaos of the night*

## SYNOPSIS

This story covers three sessions of emergency counselling over a two month period on a fortnightly basis (Service X), with a woman in her late fifties. The work, undertaken in 1996, is of a particular genre: very brief crisis work with no follow-through from the counselling team, as there were no foreseeable vacancies at that time. The intermittent service (D) is not yet fully operational, so she could not be assimilated in that way at that time.

The containment provided is of the safety net variety. From the counsellor's point of view, it is as if the patient disappears back into the general practice system, to be sustained by the GP in the normal way. From the patient's point of view, there is an opportunity to talk to someone at greater length at a time of crisis, but no more. To the receptionists, the patient is unremarkable and unremembered, just one of many who make only occasional contact and ask for little. She could have been referred to a massage therapist, but the GP chose counselling and she accepted.

Follow-up of the patient one year later, around the time of the anniversary of the bereavement, showed that, though she managed the immediate practical aspects of her crisis with the help of the GP and counsellor, she was now drinking heavily and had been for some time, at considerable cost to her health. After further help from the GP and a hospital consultant, she managed to stop drinking and is now adapting to her new life.

The example has been chosen because brief episodic work of this kind is one typical form of general practice counselling.

## REFERRAL
### The GP's story (May 1996)

Joanna is in her late fifties ... she came to see me after a bereavement which had happened some three months previously ... her husband of twenty four years had died in Los Angeles and had left her with many practical and emotional problems ... she was particularly worried because her rented flat was in her husband's name ... and she had no money and was in danger of being evicted once his death was known to the landlord .... Her husband had also run up a number of large credit card arrears when he was last in London .... Joanna was now left with having to pay these off .... She was unemployed ... on income support .... She had the remnants of a family in the south west of England but only a few good friendships in London .... I felt she was in serious trouble emotionally and practically ....

Her earlier career had been in retailing ... selling fashions in stores like Harrods ... Selfridges ... Peter Jones ... but she hadn't worked for many years because she'd devoted herself to her husband when he was in London ... caring for him ... socializing ... that sort of thing .... She has this strangely dramatic Anglo-American accent from spending a lot of time in the States ... and I think because her husband was in the film business .... I felt she was more at risk than even she realized and I wanted her seen urgently ....

> .... I felt she was more at risk than even she realized and I wanted her seen urgently ....

### The counsellor's story

I took the emergency referral one busy afternoon at a peak time of the year and rang the patient at home there and then ... the GP explained he was very worried ... but as I said to him ... I had no real feel of how the patient saw things .... With emergencies there are no Patient Request Forms and I couldn't somehow get the feel of it from him .... When I rang her however, explaining that I could only give her one or two sessions ... she was relieved and keen to come and talk things over in my next emergency slot the following week .... I decided on the basis of the GP's considerable anxiety to give her a full fifty minute session each time I saw her .... I knew I couldn't take her on more fully and felt it was going to be complex .... I thought she might need a referral elsewhere .... The following week I just had the usual emergency half-hour available and, because I had a long term

> I took the emergency referral one busy afternoon at a peak time of the year and rang the patient at home there and then ... the GP had explained he was very worried ...

case in a half-hour slot, I could use the other half-hour to give this patient a full session ... it just meant all face-to-face work that day and no admin .... The fact is we're understaffed ....

## SESSION ONE
### Joanna's story

*Told fast, with a confusing mix of real and dramatized urgency.*

Look, doll, you gotta help me ... things are going from bad to worse ... when they find out Tom's gone I'll be out on the street and I've got nothing ... nothing .... I think they suspect already because he hadn't been back for a while anyway ... he had some kinda project on ... he wanted me to go but then when I decided to stay here he said, 'Okay I'll be all right with the cat' .... He's got a place over there someone looks after ... but it took longer than he expected ... then he got ill and had to go to hospital ... chest pains ... he was in for a while .... They kept an eye on him and we used to talk on the 'phone ... he was worried about the cat then ... this cat he had over there ... sometimes I think he cared more about the cat than he did me .... We argued about that bloody cat because I felt he didn't give a damn about me ... but he just kept saying, 'I asked you to come, don't say I didn't ask you' ... (*She grinds her teeth in an alarming way, then with her mouth half open rotates her jaw from side to side in some kind of grotesque tic.*)

Well one day I got this call from his son ... we don't get on ... he hated Tom .... He just said, 'Tom's very ill ... he's in hospital in Los Angeles ... and he gave me the number .... Well I rang but I had no money ... I couldn't just get on a plane ... and I thought he'd get better anyway ... so did he. The next thing I know is he's dead from a heart attack .... There was nothing I could say .... I always thought he was coming back ... he'd always come back .... I know there was all that film world ... he loved it ... I hated it ... but he'd always come back and we'd have our London life again .... We had a nice flat here just off Regent's Park ... but now I know time is running out on that .... They keep saying to me, 'When's Tom coming back?' ... because they want the rent and I daren't tell them in case they tell me to go .... I got nowhere to go you understand? .... And I got no money ... he used to pay for everything ... cash mostly ....

But that's not all of it ... there's something else ... something really gettin' to me ... it's ... his ashes ... they're stuck in some goddam crematorium in Los Angeles and they won't let me have them .... I don't understand what the problem is .... I keep ringing and all I get is fobbed off .... I half think his son has something to do with it but I reckon that's going too far ... even tho' we don't get on .... I'll never be able to rest till his ashes come home …. (*More severe grinding of teeth and rotating of jaw.*)

Then there's money …. At one level I don't give a damn … it's him I miss … I loved him but I'm wild at him …. I want him back … ya' know what I mean? …. But it's getting worse … my last card was stopped this week … (*teeth grinding*) … all I've got now is my benefit and that doesn't even pay the rent and I can't tell them he's not coming back because, like I told you, they might throw me out …. I got no security … I just can't see a way out … thank God for my cat … and my neighbours … they've been very good to me …. Each evening they feed me …. I buy a bottle of wine and they make a pasta or something and life seems like normal again until I go home … then there's the cat …. I love her to bits … I'm nuts about her … she sits on the table and waits for me to get home …. I know it sounds daft but just to know she waits for me makes a difference …. (*Grinding teeth and rotating jaw, as if holding on very tight and trying to reason with herself.*) …. I mean he always went away … but I knew he was always coming back …. I try to do things … you know, shop and all that … but first I've got no cash and second I can't see the point …. I mean … well what do I mean? … who gives a damn? … you know what I

…. Is there anything you can do for me? …. I mean counsellors don't help with debts or anything so they? … it's just talking, isn't it? …. I don't wanna waste your time … but I gotta do something … you gotta help me … but I don't see what you can do ….

mean? …. Is there anything you can do for me, doll? …. I don't see as there's anything you can do for me …. I mean counsellors don't help with debts or anything do they? … it's just talking, isn't it? …. I don't wanna waste your time … but I gotta do something … you gotta help me … but I don't see what you can do ….

## The counsellor's story

Joanna looked like a film star in disguise. She was wearing a simple black sweater and trousers and large dark glasses … her dyed red hair was pulled back tight. She seemed at the same time someone who was very afraid and someone who was determined to cut a dash, in spite of her troubles … but on top of that, she was playing a part in a drama that wasn't her life but was rather some grotesque parody of it. Ordinary but difficult things seemed saturated with a seething menace from which she was alternately hiding and running, or so it seemed to me ….

As I listened to her story I felt breathless because she didn't stop talking … but two points touched me aside from the first impression I have just described … the ashes that she could not release … and the seeming pathos of the adults with their two cats in two capital cities, loving and hating in brittle opposition …. Her cat was at least pleased to see her … unlike her husband's American family who, according to her story at least, seemed to want to cut her out of everything … it didn't hang together somewhere but I couldn't put my finger on why not … and she was going at such a rattling pace ….

I noted she had said nothing about a will …. I also now felt and understood what the GP had said in the referral … she could easily end up living on the streets … there was something desperate about her beneath the dramatic presentation …. I could imagine her on a park bench talking to herself …. The teeth-grinding was very disturbing … because she twisted her mouth and her lips were pulled back tight to show her teeth as she moved her jaw from side to side in an anguished way … almost like an animal contorted in pain and fury … yet she had words: no job, no money and no-one close enough to give a damn ….

> …. I also now felt and understood what the GP had said in the referral … she could easily end up living on the streets … there was something desperate about her beneath the dramatic presentation …. I could imaging her on a park bench talking to herself ….

I decided finally that the GP was right to see this as an emergency …. Joanna gave an impression of raw, diffuse power not at all harnessed in her own interest … and a pathetic helplessness …. The two negated each other so she was left going round in circles … and the opposition between power and helplessness was all going into grinding her teeth …. She was trying but failing to keep up appearances … she was as she feared 'losing it' ….

I found it hard to think of how to use this clutter of thoughts and sensations but at first I say: 'It's like Tom gave you a purpose in life … now you've lost him you seem to feel you might lose everything … your home … even yourself … your sense of who you are, where you live and what your life is about' ….

*Shit, doll, she said, Don't say that to me … I don't wanna hear that …. I've gotta find a way through … or I'm done for …. I've tried applying for jobs …. I apply for about seven a week …. I get interviews … but the truth is I'm over-qualified …. I've done all the big stores, so they look at me and they think, 'What're you here for, dame? This is a kid's job.' If I could just get something …. I gotta sort out the money …. I reckon I've got a few weeks, maybe months, before they catch on that he's not coming back and if I could get a job in the meanwhile ….*

Amidst her rage, her desperation and her stagey style, I'm struck by Joanna's sense of priorities … perhaps she is a survivor … just ….

I decided quickly to work with her perception of the situation and to take an active approach encouraging 'healthy coping responses' based

---

**Figure 13.1**   Direct intervention to help with 'crisis-coping' (after Caplan 1964)

Caplan stated that practitioners could influence the choice of healthy coping responses in a crisis by:

- enlarging understanding of the situation
- supporting the expression of negative feelings
- pointing out useful avenues of further exploration
- fostering a reality framework, in order to regain a sense of how to influence outcomes through personal effort
- opening channels of communication with other helpful individuals: friends, family or professionals.

---

on my previous experience of crisis work. In my mind, I was following the work of Gerald Caplan (1964), whom I had met many years before at his annual Tavistock Clinic conferences on preventive psychiatry. I had found his work liberating, solid and full of common sense ... he seemed to me to have a wisdom based on so much experience that one felt as a clinician one could lean on him safely ....

Caplan demonstrated that different rules of therapeutic operation apply in a crisis (see Figure 13.1). Notably, one can give advice, even be directive where one would not normally do so. Instead of the patient becoming dependent, the experience of learning to survive and master what seems to be a very threatening situation gives strength that can be drawn on in future crises, and can help to create a new equilibrium. Furthermore, if one can provide 'anticipatory guidance', which means mapping the future pathway of the crisis to help the patient get a handle on it and prepare for each step, s/he can manage the worst of the helplessness with an inner map to help her/him find the way.

I arrange to see Joanna again in two weeks time ... it seems a long time away ... but I'm very busy and can only just fit her in ... some of that administration just has to wait ....

Meanwhile I give her, in a structured way, some demanding but important practical tasks to accomplish before I next see her. These tasks will act as a reminder that I'm with her in spirit, if nothing else, and give her something to hang on to. If she does them she'll benefit considerably ... as I know from my own experience of yoga training ....

So I say:

... Next time, we'll talk in detail about your debts and what you might do about them .... I have heard that these are your main worry but there's not enough time to think about them properly today, so we just have to put them on hold .... Meanwhile, I'd like you to do four practical things before the next session. If you do, they'll really help you significantly. I'm asking you:

---

**Figure 13.2** Diaphragmatic breathing and mental focusing (after Samskrti & Veda 1976)

Derived from hatha yoga, these exercises comprise the following:

- Sit poised on the edge of an upright chair or lie flat on the floor.
- Align the head, neck, back, legs and feet 'as if pulled gently but not tightly by a cord from the middle of the top of the head'.
- Consciously relax hands, legs, stomach, buttocks, shoulders, face, neck, tongue, jaw.
- Feel the contact points of the chair or the floor and allow them to support the body weight whilst remaining gently poised and elongated: 'feel the weight'.
- Breathe normally and observe the body minutely while doing so: the rise and fall of the abdomen, shoulders, chest; the feel of the breath in and out on the top lip.
- Place one hand loosely on the stomach, with thumb and first finger outlining the lower ribs and other hand on the upper chest.
- Take in this information from observing and touching: which moves most?
- Adjust the breath so that the lower hand on the stomach rises and falls significantly more than the hand on the chest (the outward sign of diaphragmatic breathing).
- Exaggerate the breath temporarily if this adjustment is difficult, in order to gain information first and then conscious control.
- Relax arms and hands on the floor again, with palms upward.
- Breathe diaphragmatically at first deeply and then more naturally, watching the breath from inside and outside while doing so.
- If the mind wanders, gently but firmly turn it back on to the movement and experience of the breathing.
- Continue for about ten minutes.
- Gently move each part of the body a little and then slowly and quietly get up.
- Avoid rushing into action afterwards; try to carry the quiet and the calm with you.
- Remember you can return to this state of body and mind at any time.

---

1. To get out of your flat every day for half an hour and to walk in the park, looking at what's around you, and breathing slowly and carefully as you walk.

2. To concentrate on eating good, regular food with water and very little alcohol. (*I guessed from her reddish, patchy face and her demeanour that she was drinking more than she acknowledged, and that this accounted for part of the dramatization.*)

3. To do diaphragmatic breathing and mental focusing for ten minutes twice a day. (*I show her how in the session, which also helps to slow her down a bit.*) This will help you stop feeling so tied up in knots, and grinding your teeth and twisting your jaw like you do. If you succeed, you'll also be able to think more clearly. (*see Figure 13.2*)

4. I also suggest you ask your solicitor for advice about how to get things moving: first, to contact the crematorium in writing to obtain a formal answer about recovering the ashes; second, to find out about the will, if there is one.

*Joanna says: You're gonna help me, I just know you're gonna find a way of helping me.*

Maybe, I say, maybe not ... we can try to work on these very difficult things but I don't know yet what will come of it ... it all depends on you ... and we haven't got long because I can't see you more than a few times just now .... What do you think?

*She goes on: Things can't get much worse .... It's worth a try .... I'll see you then ... and yes ... I'll walk .... I get your drift, doll ... I think I know what you're driving at .... I used to go to yoga once, you know .... I used to know how to breathe and all that stuff .... I will do it ... I will ....*

I speak to the GP after the first session and explain what I had in mind and that I don't know if it will work but think it's definitely worth trying and won't harm her. I also say that although I hadn't mentioned it, I wondered if she was drinking .... He thinks not but says he's worried about her. She's more depressed than she seems and very brittle ... and her stepson's treating her badly, refusing to release the ashes to her and making her feel helpless, when she already has enough to worry about with her debts and accommodation problems. The community mental health team couldn't help a great deal and anyway the patient wouldn't tolerate a referral ... or medication ....

## SESSION TWO (JUNE 1996)
### Joanna's story continued

... I did the stuff, doll ... you know ... I walked ... I looked ... I even saw some folks enjoying themselves ... that park is beautiful ... it gave me a breather ... but it doesn't sort my problems, you know? Time's running out .... I sent some more applications in and I've got another interview next week .... Oh, I did the breathing too, you know. I learned how to do that before once .... I just haven't been doing it for a while .... You're right ... it does really help ... I slept a bit better ... (*and so on*) ....

> ... I did the stuff, doll ... you know ... I walked ... I looked ... I even saw some folks enjoying themselves ... that park is beautiful ... it gave me a breather ... but it doesn't sort my problems, you know?

*She looks dire ... all dressed in black but with more surface panache with huge glasses covering her eyes ... and now dark red lips like a wound across her pasty face ....*

*I say: The problem for me is I don't know where you are ... behind those glasses and all that .... You call me doll but I get the impression it's you that feels you have to dress up like somebody's doll no matter what the human being is feeling inside ....*

They're part of the uniform .... Don't ask me to give them up .... I know if I have to I can still play the game in an interview or something .... It's all I've got left, doll .... I gotta believe I can still do it ....

*I say .... Like in here .... You decided to come for help but ... you seem to feel you have to cover up your pain and your rage at Tom for leaving you ... all that you came for ... with those glasses and that lipstick ... they're like some kind of disguise or costume ....*

... I told you ... (*crossly*) They're part of the uniform ... I always wear them ....

*... The trouble is, I go on ... you could have me thinking what's going on here is just a costume drama and behind it you, the human being, only need a little help ... as if nothing serious had happened ... no-one would think you've lost your man, might lose your home, have debts that worry you more than anything and don't have a job ... you could fool me into thinking this is not for real ... this is just a trailer and we don't need to do any real work in the short time we have .... Let's get down to it .... You wanted to focus on the money and we had to put it on hold last time ... you said it was what most worried you .... Tell me about it ....*

## The counsellor's story

She settles down at this point, loses some of her surface push and allows me to see how beaten she is. Her age was showing ... late fifties is a difficult age .... She explained to me that she owed over three thousand pounds on a series of credit cards that her husband normally paid, in addition, of course, to two months' rent: a larger sum. In another month this amount would increase by ... whatever ... then there were the ashes ... what was she going to do about the ashes? They bloody well wouldn't let her have them .... Tom's son must have a hand in all that ... she knew it .... She hadn't been to see her solicitor yet ....

I cut through with, Let's concentrate on the money today .... What's the position at your bank? They've refused to pay the cards, is that it?

*She explains that they had two banks and she's afraid to go into either. She's even started selling some small pieces of furniture ... a kitchen table ... a lamp ... but there's a limit to how far that can go ... there's not a lot anyway ....*

I guess rightly or wrongly that things are probably worse than she's telling me but not as bad as she fears ... and I wonder if she might be able to turn things round .... Then I have an idea ....

I say ... I want you to think about something ... that acting you bring in here and which I've criticized because ... it can get in the way in here and I can see how it can get on people's nerves ... but I wonder if you could try to control it a bit more? .... Could you calm down more ...

and think carefully ... and make the acting work for you instead of against you outside of here? Do you think you could harness it more, make it work for you? ....

You say you have two banks and two bank managers and two lots of debt and you're frightened to go into either bank .... Yet you tell me you've been in business, you know how to sell things ... including yourself .... Banks are only businesses after all ... if they think you're a loser they won't invest in you; if they think you're still thinking and have a future they might believe in you (or at least hold fire) if you could convince them it was worth it ....

*... I don't want to be a loser ....*

Well, imagine for a moment that I'm one of these two bank managers and you come into my office to persuade me to take on all your credit card debts (which are at high rates of interest) in exchange for a bank loan (at a lower rate of interest) which you'll start to pay off once you get your job and have paid off the rent that's owed. You'll have to get the interest rates clear first, of course .... Then explain the situation to me as the bank manager, clearly, firmly and quietly, without too much of that drama ... it puts people off ... so you have several interviews coming up ... you're newly widowed ... you just need a little time to put your affairs in order and this is one more step to help turn things round ... do you get the idea? .... Remember how you felt on the walk in the park and when you were doing the breathing? ... use that ... make it work for you ....

*... Doll, I don't know I can do it .... I never deal with banks .... They scare me ... always have ... that's why Tom did everything ....*

I sense nevertheless that she's coming along with me and thinking about it in an intrigued sort of way ... but she needs more help with the split inside her between her helplessness and that raw power that seems to be doing nothing useful ....

I say ... she's shown me the different sides of herself and I'm going to label them now ... rather rudely ... as a way of making things clearer .... I want you to hold inside that 'fractured widow' part of yourself who's too frightened and helpless to go in to the bank ... and the 'unconvincing actress' that I've warned you about ... and I want you to show me the lady, the woman, the adult part of you who can think and plan and is determined to take control of her life again ... having been left in a hole .... But it's no good looking like an actress ... it's not convincing ... everyone sees through that ... the fact is you really are a woman, a wife who's trying to get her life back, to get back in control, that is completely reasonable and true ... you don't *need* to act it ... you have a choice ... if you recognize that you can do it ....

*... I'm so angry ... (grinding her teeth for the first time that day) ... so angry ... how could he leave me in this mess? ....*

... But he did ... it seems ... and you're the only one who's going to get you out of it, and you know that ... but you're so furious it's hard to accept that now only you can sort it out ... so how about trying to turn things round with those bank managers? Why, for example, not interview both of them? You say you've been to lots of interviews of late but never get the jobs ... and it gets you down being on the end of the interviews all the time .... How about you turn things around and you go and interview each of them and see which one treats you better? You could aim to have all that credit card debt turned into a bank loan, which you agree to start repaying only when you get work and have got your rent sorted out. You ought to be able to get one of those bank managers on your side .... Take control .... It's one of the things you could have some control over ... and the worst they could do is turn you down or laugh at you and even then you wouldn't in fact be any worse off than you are now ... but you'd have to be ready for that .... Could you take it, do you think? .... Or would it make you feel even worse?

There was a pause and she looks quieter ... as if she's weighing up the options. Her jaw's going like before but silently. I can see she's thinking ....

*You are a doll .... I can see it could go wrong .... I get your drift about the acting bit but I feel better just at the thought of doing something for me, something positive .... I could do it ... I know I could do it .... I know one of 'em a bit anyway .... I'll do it ... even if I fail ... it'd make me feel better just to try .... I'll do it ... but can I see you again?*

## THIRD AND FINAL SESSION

*Two weeks later she comes back, still in the dark glasses but this time in a suit and so city-elegant I hardly recognize her. Another act perhaps, but more convincing and more functional, and therefore more positive ....*

### Joanna's story continued

*As she comes into the room, she walks across to me and gives me a big kiss on the cheek ....*

Doll ... he's thinking about it ... he's gonna let me know ... he said they didn't realize Tom was dead ... no-one had told them ... and I never thought to .... And I got two interviews next week ... something's gonna come up, I know it is .... I just feel so much better even though I'm so damned angry (*grinding her teeth still*). I can't forgive him for leaving me in this mess, but perhaps I can find my way out of it .... I've got good neighbours you know ... they don't tell the landlord Tom's not coming back ... and we eat most evenings ... but I'm so angry I still wanna kill someone (*grinding teeth and rotating jaw again*) .... I never thought it would come to this ... how could he leave me like this? .... It's years since I worked seriously ... because I just used to look after him when he came home .... He had been ill before ... like with his heart ... so we had to be careful but I used to spoil him ... get him nice things .... He was my life ... like you said ... the shit ... now he does this to me ... no provision whatever .... God knows what was in the will .... I couldn't even go to the funeral .... It was in LA .... I had no money and all those movie people were gonna be there and I didn't wanna see them anyway ... what we had we had and we had it for a long time ... over twenty years .... I still don't know if there was a will ... we never discussed anything like that ... and I don't trust that son of his to let me know even though he knows what we had ... in time I suppose the solicitors will ....

*I say ... The trouble is ... there's lots more to do .... I know it and you know it but as you also know we're out of time. This is the last emergency session available just now and I understand from Dr Yo that you don't want to go any- where else .... And we've only just begun to scratch the surface .... I notice you're still doing that teeth-grinding ... you feel murderous and you say you want to kill someone ... if Tom's dead then his son is number two ... I could be number three ... for entering your life and then leaving it so quickly ... for having done so little when you need so much ... or you could make yourself number three of course ... you must know we're worried about that too ....*

I knew that, doll ... you laid it on the line and hell, I didn't know if it would make any difference at all to see you .... It could've made things worse ... instead I feel I've got something back .... It's hard to explain and things will probably get worse again but for now I feel I've got something to stay alive for ... and it's not just the cat .... There's lots to do ... I can see that now ... and I'm still walking every day .... I make myself ... and I breathe properly ... some o' the time anyway .... Maybe I'll see you again some time but for now thanks ... a real big thanks .... You got hold o' something I thought I'd lost ....

## The counsellor's story continued

This was a piece of work with lots of limitations. It was all I could do in the time. I knew Joanna was less at risk at the end of these three ses- sions than at the beginning, but she was still at risk, and I had to make that explicit so she would know we knew .... I was impressed that she managed to get to the bank manager and relieved that he hadn't turned her down immediately ... taking charge like that did seem to have helped .... I was also sure that if she kept walking, and even did the diaphragmatic breathing for short periods of time, she would break the cycle of hyperventilation and dramatization in which she trapped herself .... I hadn't taken up the drinking and I should have done .... I was pretty sure of it even if the GP wasn't ... on the plus side although she was so dramatic she did have a positive effect on people as well ... on me, the GP, the bank manager, her neighbour ... this augured well.

I felt very doubtful about the work but I had to move on, like a GP in some ways. Yet to be so directive can make one feel one is going out on a limb, whatever the precedents – and I felt they were good ones. Working like that felt quite natural at the time but after each of the sessions I had misgivings .... I realized I should have tackled the possible drinking more clearly ... but I didn't ... it was one of those occasions though when Caplan's specific theory combined with stress management skills drawn from yoga, helped me to find a way of responding and it did seem to have provided her with a safety net ... not only that ... if I had tried to get her to accept a referral somewhere else she would have had to wait and she probably would not have got there in the state she was in ....

## ONE YEAR LATER
### The GP's story continued

Joanna was better for a while. She pulled out of her trough and I felt less worried about her and then I didn't see her for a long time .... Then I got a note to say she'd been admitted to hospital after some internal bleeding ... it was associated with heavy drinking ... they'd given her an ultimatum .... After that she stopped and the hospital consultant has been going on seeing her periodically as an outpatient. His last letter said what a pleasant woman she was and how hard she had worked to pull out of it ... that's unusual for a consultant to write like that ... she's still at her flat ... but I haven't seen her for a while .... I think it was the anniversary of her husband's death that tipped her over the edge again ....

## IN CONCLUSION ...

### Containment

- The patient was provided with a combination of the safety net and the transformative forms of containment by the counsellor, the former to support her and to try and keep the lid on and help her to cope.
- Crisis intervention theory indicates that directive work can

provide a safety net and can sometimes be transformative in the longer term (Caplan 1964).

• Stress management skills of diaphragmatic breathing and mental focusing, taught in the first session, allowed enough entry into the patient's mind to do some work which would otherwise probably have been impossible.

## Multi-professional teamwork

• GP and counsellor worked together, but the patient did not want any other interventions.

• The patient was able, with help, to gain the support of her bank manager (Caplan's 'helpful other'), and later the hospital consultant, in addition to the GP and counsellor.

## Outcomes

• Indeterminate: the patient may have been given a breathing space through the sessions, but the failure to take up her drinking as another form of slow suicide may have been critical.

• The clinical question is whether the counsellor
— colluded with the patient's defence of dramatization by using role play
— or turned it to good effect, helping the patient to achieve a temporary respite from one of her most worrying problems and to achieve more perspective on the others.

## Postmodernism

• Global city: the contest for the patient's husband's ashes took place across two large cities.

• Banalization: this patient (and, by her account, her husband too) made superficial dramas out of serious, even life and death, issues: his illness, the ashes, the debts, the rent/landlord problem, the counselling session used as a stage set. Ordinary but serious real life problems were disguised as extraordinary dramas.

• Impact of technology on life: the patient seemed to inhabit a virtual world of the gangster movie, and to use its emotional and verbal language: her 'doll/moll' construct, and the ubiquitous atmosphere of menace.

• Superficial language games: the languages of the gangster movie, of the cosy London flat life with cats, of the 'competent retailer', of the 'fractured widow' and the 'woman about town' were used interchangeably, and supported by different costumes and different make-up, like different parts in a drama, reflecting alienation between different internal parts of the self, exacerbated by the fragmenting pressures of life in the inner city.

# 14

# The leaving

*Marilyn Pietroni**

Upon the maple leaves The dew shines red, But on the lotus blossom It has the pale transparence of tears.

Amy Lowell, Circumstance in *Imagist poetry*

---

## SYNOPSIS

This chapter describes fortnightly work over a ten month period with a young English woman in her thirties, who presented with severe phobic problems and is now making a good recovery. The initial brief work of ten fortnightly sessions over twenty weeks (Service C) was extended exceptionally, with the GPs agreement, to twenty sessions because the patient was doing so well. Her mental state and financial position made it difficult to transfer her to another counsellor or psychotherapist and, as it was her first time of seeking help, it was a unique opportunity to save resources in the longer term. The story is told in three parts: early work, middle work and present work.The form of containment provided is transformative. The counselling method is primarily cognitive-behavioural, although supervision provided a psychodynamic perspective.

---

## EARLY WORK

## The GP's story (July 1997)

*Referral*

*Dr Anagha Shah, though not a partner, is now an appointed member of the GP team in the practice, having been a regular locum for many years. She remembered the referral well ....*

... It was about a year ago that I first met her here ... she was a new patient ... and it was her first time here .... I recall that she was a really

---

*Romayne Jesty, the third member of our counselling team, provided the counselling viewpoint in a series of interviews with the author and approved the final manuscript.

beautiful girl ... but nervous ... tense ... very timid ... she told me it had been difficult to come and make the first move .... I remember her words: 'I'm suffering from agoraphobia and I've had it for as long as I can remember' .... She actually used that word ... and she told me how it was very difficult to get out and that she was confined to home .... She was unemployed and she said it was difficult to get out to get her benefits too ....

I remember thinking this girl can be helped ... definitely .... Counselling will do something for her ... she was very genuine and it was so severe ... on a nought to five severity scale where five is high she would be about four ... she couldn't go out and do any daily things ... although she wasn't depressed as such ....

We don't see many people like that here ... you do in psychiatry but she needed a psychological approach not a psychiatric one .... I thought it would open her out a bit and that she might get some real benefit from a cognitive approach ... that's what the research suggests .... Her only support at that time was her employer ... there were no friends or family involved ... she'd lost the links when she stopped going out to work and was very disappointed in her family ... and she felt they were disappointed in her too ....

> I remember thinking this girl can be helped ... definitely .... Counselling will do something for her ... she was very genuine and it was so severe ... on a nought to five severity scale ... where five is high ... she would be about four ... she couldn't go out and do any daily things ... although she wasn't depressed as such ....

I warmed to her ... she had a real problem that could really be helped .... I said that we could consider other treatment and I laid out the options to her with medication as a last resort .... Then as we are meant to do ... I gave her the counselling leaflet and sent her away and asked her to come back and let me know what she thought about it .... She came back the next week and I thought she was motivated for change and ready to work ....

It makes extra work for the GPs to do it that way ... you know with these two appointments before making a referral to the counsellors ... but I understand the reasons and I know the DNAs have dropped dramatically since we introduced the new system .... All that saves counselling resources ... and ensures more patients have access ... and I do feel we need more counselling here ... with it being the inner city and all that that implies ....

### The referral form

Francesca Delamere registered June 1997. Age 31. Seen three times. Severe agoraphobia, shaking, dizziness. Unemployed: income support.

Little contact with own family. No previous counselling or psychotherapy. First time seeking help. Feels she is a disappointment to her parents.

## The counsellor's response

I had a sinking feeling because this patient clearly had a deep and long term problem. It may be impossible to assess and work with this degree of disturbance in the time available. Perhaps she should be referred on to a more specialist agency, like the Tavistock Clinic? I know she'll need a lot of help to get there, however, and to manage their assessment system, so perhaps she'll need to be seen here at MHC first anyway .... Then again, I wonder if she'll ever get here?

> I had a sinking feeling because this patient had a deep and long term problem.

There was a delay of eight weeks before Francesca was seen because she went to stay in a friend's empty house to do some decorating for six weeks ... it was the sort of indoors work that she could manage, and she needed the money ....

## EARLY WORK

### The patient's story

*Francesca was crouched in a corner in the waiting room ... all dressed in black and accompanied by an older man who seemed to be protecting her in some way as she waited .... There was a tension in the way she held herself ... and she had wide, frightened eyes .... She was tall, slim and strikingly beautiful, with a long cascade of black hair .... She followed me to the room and spoke straight away but haltingly ... when I asked if it was difficult to get to the health centre ....*

> ... I live alone ... and I've been like this ... agoraphobic ... for as long as I can remember .... I haven't seen my family for years ....

My boss came with me ... but I live alone ... and I've been like this ... agoraphobic ... for as long as I can remember .... I haven't seen my family for years .... 'My family', I call them ... but I think they're disappointed with me .... They live in the country .... At school I felt like this too ... afraid of people I mean .... I did work from home for a while but the business went bust .... I was a secretary .... I was working from home because my boss said I could ... that was four years ago ... and things have been very bad since then ... and I'm getting worse .... I've left things ... but the longer I wait the worse it gets .... I'm so anxious I feel sick, physically sick .... My boss has been very good though ... that was him in the waiting room ... I repay him by doing little chores ... you know ... washing and ironing, mending sometimes ... and when I do manage to go out I do the shopping ....

*(She laughed mirthlessly)* ....

I feel I'm the only person in the world with this problem ... do you know of anyone who has got better from it? .... I wish there hadn't been this delay in seeing you but I had to go away because I was offered a job doing some decorating for a friend and I needed the money badly ... it's one of the things I can do ... my mother taught me ... and it means I can stay in and do it, you see ... once I get over the journey problem ....

*When invited to say a little more about her family background since she had herself alluded to it earlier she responded as follows* ....

I know it all began a long time ago .... There was no socializing at home ... my mother was ... is rather ... a very houseproud person ... no-one was allowed to visit our house unless she had cleaned it from top to bottom ... very thoroughly ... so we led rather solitary lives ... there were three of us besides my mother and father ... my older brother's a lawyer now and my sister's younger ... we don't see each other ... any of us ....

*She continued in this halting but illuminating way* ....

... My father was different ... but then he had this terrible accident when I was about twelve ... he was in a car crash and he was nearly killed but ended up losing both of his legs ... so I was sent off to boarding school .... I would try and stay there at weekends pretending that I'd been asked out by someone else ... sometimes I did go with a friend and I found other families were quite different ... relaxed ... friendly .... They dressed differently too .... I wore my school uniform all the time in the end because it made me like the other girls ... but my mother always dressed me in bright colours ... cotton dresses with puffed sleeves ... that sort of thing ... everything ironed beautifully ... but it just wasn't what other people wore and I felt very awkward .... I knew we were different somehow but I didn't know why ....

My father had always had affairs ... so after the accident my mother used to taunt him ... she'd say, 'You can't go anywhere else now, can you?' .... So there we all were ... shut up together and no-one coming in ... it was pretty difficult and I'm sure it's got something to do with my agoraphobia ... it's not surprising that I can't go out ... being frightened all the time ... feeling different and everything ....

*So far I felt Francesca had begun to give a fairly clear picture of her problems and how she had come to understand them ... and I decided to let her continue to help me figure out what was going on and how to respond .... I was pleased she had come and now here she seemed ready to start work ... but at this point*

*I had no clear idea of what I was going to say or do ... but the session was going better than I had expected ....*

... When I got older I had a lot more problems with my mother ... she wrote me a letter when I was twenty five accusing me of being a flirt and shameless and that sort of thing ... and then she just went on sending the same letter over and over .... I was so upset ... so angry too ... because it wasn't true .... I used to wear big shapeless sweaters and that sort of thing ... up till then ... but that letter had a big effect on me .... I changed after that really .... I started wearing tight clothes and black ... more tailored things ... smarter .... I wanted to get away and on with my own life ... and for a while it worked .... I met a man and had a relationship that went on for a few years ... but then he wanted to marry me and I knew I couldn't ... so we split up ... but we're still in touch ... he helps me by giving me bits of work to do at home sometimes ....

*I found myself thinking, So she has had a fuller life at some point and now it has become restricted again .... I wonder why? ....*

Now I go out very rarely ... once a week I get my benefits and go shopping .... I have to wear sunglasses ... summer's such a difficult time because everyone undresses ... if you see what I mean ... but I never go anywhere without my leather coat and bag .... My boss ... that's what I call him ... teases me about it ... but I can't go without them ... when I'm wearing summer clothes I feel so exposed ... and there always seem to be more people about too .... I wish I could be invisible ... I really do ....

....I wish I could be invisible ... I really do ....

## The counsellor's story

I felt straight away that I had to let Francesca tell her story in her own way .... I knew it must have been a struggle for her to get here at all .... I recognized that she had taken herself off to do the decorating just when the sessions were going to be offered but I didn't want to make the beginning too tough for her by starting in on this issue .... So I just noted how tightly she controlled her contacts and her comings and goings, just like her mother .... She had such a striking presence but seemed so fragile ... she made me think of a bygone romantic age ... pre-raphaelite perhaps ... there was something nostalgic in her face .... I listened hard as she paused to explain how she wished she could make herself invisible when she went out ... it was then that I began to recognize that this fantasy-wish could be used to help her get out more ....

... So I decided to start straight in on her symptoms with a fairly active directive approach .... I could then find out how far she could

... So I decided to start straight in on her symptoms with a fairly active directive approach .... I could then find out how far she could work with me and what might be possible in the short time we were going to have together .... work with me and what might be possible in the short time we were going to have together .... I had experience of using active imagination strategies for managing anxiety from my training in person-centred therapy and I am currently an apprentice in one of the cognitive-analytical therapy schemes in central London, so my approach is somewhat different from my colleagues.

So when Francesca said she wished she could be invisible ... I suggested to her that perhaps she could try a 'strategy' to imagine actively that she was invisible ... to tell herself before she goes out, 'I am invisible. Nobody notices me. I am invisible. Nobody notices me.' Like a mantra that she could repeat each time before leaving the house .... Something to have in her mind or even say aloud to herself when the anxiety began to increase each time just before she goes out. 'I am invisible. Nobody notices me. I am invisible. Nobody notices me.' I also suggested that she prepare the ground for this mantra by telling herself, 'People are too interested in their own lives to be looking at me.'

I wondered how she would take to these ideas ... and was aware that she might feel it was rather odd ... but I knew it could work if she could 'allow it in' ... and I didn't feel I could work directly with that difficult history in the time available without losing her ... time was of the essence ... and if she was unable to start work quickly she might not come back ... also we have a practice of seeing whether a patient can respond to a specific intervention in the first assessment session ... to see if they can use further sessions ... it's one of our assessment criteria ....

Francesca looked at me for a while, said she did feel less visible when wearing her sunglasses and that she felt she could try repeating the bit about 'People are too interested in their own lives to notice me' ... she also said, 'When I'm out I could walk really fast to start with, as well .... I find that helps .... I'm not sure about the rest but I'll try' ....

When I enquired what Francesca did alone at home all the time ... she explained that she reads a lot and spends time writing short stories ... she also sews and embroiders .... She gave me the impression of living in a closed ... almost Victorian existence that was closer than she wanted to admit to her mother's way of doing things ....

## MIDDLE WORK

*Francesca was able to use the mantra and it worked for her. She was surprised that it had definitely helped her to feel less anxious now when she went out. However, so far she had not increased her outings beyond the original once a week for necessities. Nevertheless, she was attending her fortnightly sessions regularly, and was now showing signs of wanting to make more changes ....*

## The patient's story continued

*Princess Diana had just been killed in a car crash and Francesca looked on with envy because Diana's brother had spoken up for her ... her family appeared to support her ....*

... She was so loved .... I wish it could have been like that for me but it wasn't .... I was thrown out .... I'm not going to contact my sister again ... she doesn't care about me .... I've just got to get out more .... I need you to help me ... it's all very well my staying home and typing things for my friend but I can't go on like this for ever ... and when the housing benefit people come I feel terrified .... I just can't open the door ... I hide ... unless I've just cleaned everything ... then it's a bit easier ... just like my mother .... I know what you're thinking ....

> ... it's all very well my staying home and typing things for my friend but I can't go on like this for ever ... and when the housing benefit people come I feel terrified ... I just can't open the door .... I hide ...

## The counsellor's story continued

I commented that she did indeed seem to feel very alone with her fear ... perhaps having taken one step to control it, which had worked, she could take things a step further? ... use a new strategy? She'd mentioned she liked dogs and that a neighbour had a dog that was rarely taken out ... why not take the dog with her and go for a walk beyond the shops into the park? .... We discussed the idea a little ... building it on to the work we had done before ... with the mantra ... which I suggested she continue to use .... I pointed out that going with a dog saved her from feeling alone but gave her a certain anonymity ... and it protected her from having to go with another person .... The emphasis was on taking things forward one step at a time ... working with the grain of her problems but pushing her forward all the time ....

Francesca took up this new strategy and in the next two weeks had been to the park twice each week .... She'd also managed when the housing benefit people came ... even if she did have to clean the flat first ... the problem was that they didn't come when they'd said they would ... so she'd cleaned for nothing ... then the next week they'd arrived when she wasn't expecting them ... but she'd been able to let them in and talked to them for ten minutes .... She'd also telephoned the friend she'd done the decorating for to get some more recommendations for indoor work to help with her financial situation ....

After this new step, her boss went away and she felt unable to continue making changes for a while ... she stayed in for two weeks without even venturing to the launderette ... but when he returned she resumed her push for progress .... I didn't take up this relationship but I noted it ....

I decided simply to press on ... and suggested to her that as she'd already made some progress over going out, the next step should be to work on her problem about allowing people in to her home ... perhaps she could ask a friend to her home for tea?

At this point in the session she visibly shook ... as if I'd chosen to confront her worst fear ... but she agreed to try and made it clear she'd like to succeed .... She volunteered also that there was an exhibition that she very much wanted to see ... a collection of fairy paintings ... at the Hayward ....

A few weeks later she'd been unable to get to the gallery but had taken up my suggestion to have friends to her flat and had managed to do so on two occasions ... a major step forward .... These were potentially 'real friends' she explained ... not just the people associated with her past work .... She'd had to clean a lot but it didn't seem to bother her so much because it was for visits that she really wanted to make possible .... She'd also managed to resume walking the dog twice a week .... The new progress excited her and seemed to give her renewed determination to break out of her self-imposed prison ... although she was still visibly ... shaky in the sessions.

Next I suggested that she start to take the dog out every day, to normalize things ... to prove to herself that she could go out every day just like other people .... Again she seemed stressed at the idea but acknowledged that being able to go out every day had been one of her own targets ....

By the next session in two weeks time, she'd been out every day ... for the first time she began to talk about having a future again .... She said she would like three things: to run her own business from home ... to have a relationship with a man ... and to have a couple of close friends .... We were approaching Christmas and I said it sounded like three Christmas wishes with the suggestion of some New Year's resolutions ... in other words a plan for more work ....

---

**Figure 14.1**  Strategies for behavioural change

- The 'mantra' to help her manage her anxiety about going out.
- Taking the neighbour's dog with her twice a week.
- Asking a friend home for tea.
- Taking the dog out every day.

## The supervisor's story

The patient and counsellor are obviously doing well together ... and the GPs agree about extending the counselling input ... but there are always new problems associated with moving away from very brief work without having the resources to move into the long term ... how to manage dependency ... how to set a new frame clearly ... how to continue to manage negative and positive transference ... often therapeutic progress of the kind Francesca made is followed by a regression, known in the literature as a negative therapeutic reaction (Freud 1923) (Figure 14.2). Partly this is because successful change brings the idea of ending the sessions, so the loss of the counsellor or therapist is felt to be nearer, and there is a wish to delay that loss or put it off altogether. At an unconscious level, there may also be resentment at giving the counsellor the pleasure of a satisfactory conclusion, and some envy of their pleasure and success ... accompanied by an unconscious wish to spoil it all by returning to square one (Horney 1936).

I discuss with the counsellor the advantages and disadvantages of extending the work .... Francesca's progress is definite but fragile and we agree she might slip back and feel 'thrown out' if the work ends at ten sessions as previously planned .... She's also likely to have major problems not only about seeing someone new but also about travelling to another agency ... and she has no money to pay privately in order to see someone near her home ....

The option of continuing seems to make sense all round so we discussed it with the GPs in our next meeting with them ....

They've been impressed at the changes in her so far and support our recommendation for a further ten fortnightly sessions .... They describe her as 'more ordinary, less estranged' and generally 'looser and easier'. The receptionists on the other hand have little to say about

---

**Figure 14.2** Negative therapeutic reaction (from Freud 1923, pp. 49–52)

There are certain people who behave in a quite peculiar fashion [...] When one speaks hopefully to them or expresses satisfaction with the progress of treatment, they show signs of discontent and their condition invariably becomes worse. One begins by regarding this as defiance and as an attempt to prove their superiority [...] but later one comes to take a deeper and juster view. One becomes convinced, not only that such people cannot endure any praise or appreciation, but that they react inversely to the progress of the treatment [...] they get worse during the treatment instead of getting better. They exhibit what is known as a 'negative therapeutic reaction'. There is no doubt that there is something in these people that sets itself against their recovery, and its approach is dreaded as though it were a danger [...] In the end we come to see that we are dealing with [...] a sense of guilt, which is finding its satisfaction in the illness and refuses to give up the punishment of suffering.

her … she seems invisible to them … which perhaps reflects how much work there still is to do ….

## The receptionist's story

*Just how successful Francesca is at making herself invisible, in spite of her dramatic looks, is borne out by what the receptionist has to say ….*

I know you've seen this patient for a while now because I recognize her name from the appointment list but I just cannot remember her …. I've asked the others too and they all say the same thing … they know her name but they cannot place her at all …. I'll look out for her next time she's in … Friday, isn't it? ….

*One week later.*

… Strange … she's such a beautiful girl … a striking girl … but I'd never seen her before, I swear it … she sits hidden behind the alcove over there … outside the practice waiting room … in the lobby … and she looks out round the corner to see if Romayne is coming … nervous like … very timid … she doesn't come in to the desk at all to say she's here … so it's not surprising we don't really know her …. I thought that when I saw her I'd say, 'Oh, that's who she is' … but not at all …. I really don't know her …. That's really unusual here …. I know nearly all the patients because I've been here since the practice opened all those years ago … and she's got that beautiful black hair … very long ….

> … she doesn't come in to the desk at all to say she's here … so it's not surprising we don't really know her …

## The GP's story continued

Well, I referred her in July 1997, and the only other contact I've had with her was in August that year when she came in saying it was still difficult to get to the benefits office and would I write her a letter so she could get it sent direct and I did …. I know that one might want to keep the pressure on her to go out … but I didn't think it was the time to do that …. I felt she needed our support most of all … to feel that we were behind her … she was so fragile and alone ….

She came in saying that counselling was proving tremendously helpful … and she was looking brighter and was much more interactive …. I could see for myself the benefit she was getting … but I saw that she still had difficulties and that it would take a long time … as I put in my letter to them here on the file … 'inevitably a long slow process' …. I thought if we pushed things, she just might regress and it would spoil everything so I talked to Romayne and sent the letter …. I've had no other contact with her at all apart from that ….

Looking back on it ... and as I discussed with her ... my other options were to send her to the district psychologist or as a very last resort drugs .... I think if we hadn't helped her, she'd have been stuck on her own in her own little world and we wouldn't have seen any more of her until much later on ... years later ... when some major crisis would have occurred ... then she'd have been a big drain on NHS resources at that stage .... I think the counselling features very strongly here at MHC as part of the integrated health and healing approach that we use .... I wish we had more of it .... I try to ration my referrals and find other ways of responding because we just don't have enough ....

## CURRENT WORK

### The counsellor's story continued

Francesca returned from the Christmas break saying that although she had felt lonely she had been able to manage much better than usual and she felt less fearful .... She explained that she felt 'more normal' having realized that it doesn't matter how other people view her if she's happy in herself .... It seemed like a major discovery ... a liberation ... to me it seemed she'd begun to internalize our earlier work ... taking it to a deeper level .... Soon after that she went to an exhibition although she'd missed the one at the Hayward ... and she loved it .... 'London's empty in winter,' she explained .... She'd also spontaneously gone into a second-hand book shop and felt that it was the sort of place that she could work ... 'somewhere dark and often empty' .... It was as if she was accepting that she'd always have limitations on what felt possible ... but also felt she could find a 'good enough' life within those limitations ....

### The supervisor's story continued

In the supervision I'd listened and watched with some awe and not a little anxiety about a way of working that was so different from my own ... for example, the strategy about imagining that she was invisible had seemed to go against all psychodynamic principles about working on defences in order to explore and understand underlying fantasies or anxieties ... and there was, as yet, very little work by the counsellor on the here-and-now or transference aspects ... linked to successful outcomes by Malan's extensive brief psychotherapy research (see Figure 14.3). This involves the way the relationship with the counsellor replicates

In the supervision I'd listen and watched with some awe and not a little anxiety about the way of working that was so different from my own ...

---

**Figure 14.3** Negative transference and outcomes (from Malan 1976, p. 52)

The aspects of technique studied [...] consisted essentially of the relation between outcome [...] and various aspects of transference interpretation [...] It emerged that those therapies tended to be successful in which:

- transference arose early
- the negative transference was thoroughly interpreted
- the link was made between the transference and the relation to parents
- the patient was able to work through grief and anger about termination.

---

other relationships in the patient's life, or shows through behaviour and its emotional impact on the counsellor, what is unconsciously being brought for attention ....

I did have some experience of being on the receiving end of very different ways of working, however, and I knew I had to suspend judgements based merely on a difference between my way of working and this counsellor's .... I also knew the literature showed that a more cognitive-behavioural approach (see Figure 14.4) worked well with phobic patients (Anderson & Hasler 1979) .... And, most important of all ... the evidence from the GPs, the patient herself and the counsellor was that this patient was visibly gaining from the counselling ... and was continuing to work .... Nevertheless, I believed the transference relationship would have to be worked through and I felt we must be in for a rough time at some point because it was all going too well ....

Just after the offer of increased sessions was made, the counsellor came to supervision in a very worried state ....

## The counsellor's story continued

I'm so worried ... she's going backwards again ... she came to the last session very depressed ... bleak ... and she'd had this awful dream about her family .... It was as if she'd never had plans for the future ... she was crying and she said although she'd walked the dog the same as usual she was frightened because the last time she'd felt as depressed as this it lasted a long time .... She'd been unable to watch TV ... and had hardly read anything either .... However ... she'd had this strange dream ... I'm not sure what it means ....

## The patient's story continued

... I had this dream .... I went to visit my old family home ... every room was there just as it used to be ... everything was in its place ... I walked upstairs and went to my old bedroom where the book shelves held all the books I had when I was a child .... Then I heard my family

> **Figure 14.4**   Cognitive-behavioural approach (Keithley & Marsh 1995, p. 172)
>
> Cognitive-behavioural approaches include:
> - analyzing the patterns of events, thoughts and feelings
> - identifying where the possibilities for change are in these patterns
> - exploring the options with the client
> - helping the client to learn techniques to identify beliefs or irrational thought processes in order to change feelings
> - development of behavioural techniques and skills to change feelings.

talking downstairs and I realized they were still there ... and still carrying on as if I'd never existed ... as if I was unimportant to them ... and I felt very sad ....

A strange thing was that there were leaves everywhere ... all over the stairs and in my room .... I felt so lonely ... yet I was afraid that my mother would come ....

*She continued with further associations to the dream ....*

When I was little I used to go and stay in my grandmother's house in the country with my brother ... we used to go out walking every day ... and I loved it there .... The terrible thing was that afterwards ... when we came home ... my mother used to make awful remarks about my grandmother .... It was as if she were teaching us to hate her .... Now I come to think about it ... I think my mother was jealous every time I was happy ... but she used to imagine I had a much busier ... much happier life than I actually did ....

## The counsellor's story continued

As Francesca told the story of her dream and her precious holiday times with her grandmother ... a good female figure in her life ... it seemed to me she was revisiting her childhood home as if she were a ghost who could revisit and see things that she hadn't seen before ....

I simply said to her, 'It sounds ghostly .... I wonder what the leaves mean?' .... She said she didn't know but she had this feeling when she woke up that her mother was somehow more real ... more ordinary ....

I said that perhaps ... if it was at last possible to revisit ... it might also be possible to leave in a new way ... particularly to leave the bad things behind and find some of the good ones again ....

## The supervisor's story continued

The counsellor here was feeling out of her depth at first because of the sudden seeming regression of the patient and the powerful dream material .... I on the other hand ... seeing things from a psychodynamic point of view ... had been waiting and hoping for something like this ... and having the benefit of more distance from the impact of the patient ... I felt relieved at the turbulence both in the transference in the session and in the dream, because its nature signalled that real or inner change was indeed occurring ....

I nevertheless had a knot in my stomach because the counsellor was very worried ... and the patient was a worrying patient ... but it was a moment when the two counselling approaches, cognitive and psychodynamic, seemed to come together and proved complementary ....

I was able to confirm that the regression and depression in the session ... and in the dream ... were a healthy part of letting go of some aspects of the past. I confirmed the counsellor's intuitive sense that Francesca was taking her leave of her family inside herself in a new way .... I suggested that the leaves everywhere in the dream signalled that preoccupation with 'leaving' her family in a new way ... putting them into a different perspective ... and that she was beginning to realize that one day soon she would have to take leave of the counsellor too and get on with her life as best she could ... unless she could become strong enough to contemplate some longer term help from elsewhere ... the trouble was that this recognition also meant that she had to face the end of her sessions and the loss of her relationship with the counsellor ... at an unconscious level the only solution to this threat was to regress so that she would have to continue ... the paradox that promotes negative therapeutic reaction. (See Figure 14.2.)

A very fruitful two-way discussion in supervision preceded a period when the counsellor adapted her approach to the changes in Francesca, started to work more in the here-and-now and also toughened up ....

## The counsellor's story continued

I felt relieved that my supervisor was not as alarmed by Francesca's new depression as I was ... that had been a terrible session for me when I thought it was all coming unravelled ... but I was intrigued by the idea that the leaves in the dream ... which were a puzzle to me ... might link up with my idea that she was revisiting her family to leave them in a new way ... inside herself ... it was exciting to make a connection like that .... So this important session seemed to signal a turning point after all ... but it was followed

> I felt relieved that my supervisor was not as alarmed by Francesca's new depression as I was ... that had been a terrible session for me when I thought it was all coming unravelled ...

by some particularly difficult life event which she managed effectively beyond all of our expectations ....

The boss who had been so good to her and had brought her to her first session, had signed her name on a lease for a flat without her permission .... He had forged her signature and then told her about it afterwards. He was the one she had worked for and she owed him a lot since then ... but not this much .... She was furious and rang the bank to tell them she knew nothing about the lease and was not intending to pursue it .... As a result, her boss had now walked out of her life .... 'I'm worth more than that, aren't I?' she said to me ....

After this she counted up the people left in her life: 'the cleaning lady in the flats, the Tesco check-out girl, the DSS benefits people, me and the dog lady' ... although she only ever passes a few words with them anyway .... Now she declared she was ready to have another go ... to find a friend, a real friend not associated with work ... the problem was where to meet them ... but she must find a real friend now that she was able to invite them to her home .... In the same session she also announced that she wanted to visit the National Film Theatre ... for the first time for years ... because she loves film and she can now just about imagine walking across Hungerford Bridge, which would allow her to avoid the tube ....

This turbulent but steady progress has continued ... there have been more sessions which she began with feelings of uselessness ... but I gradually began to take a tougher and more humorous approach ... helping her to establish more reflective distance on her problems and to recognize their recurring pattern .... For example, one day she came in talking about men shouting after her in the street ... on the one hand she was wanting to introduce the subject of her sexuality which she had so far avoided ... on the other she was turning something everyday into a drama and then reacting to it .... She also went on in a repetitive way about not eating much that week and I commented somewhat abruptly ....

'Well, I don't suppose it's terminal ... you know you remind me at times of the Snow Queen; sometimes you have a kind of frozen beauty but you keep everyone at a distance including me .... It's as if were you to allow me to touch your feelings more, you might melt and turn out to be an ordinary woman more like me and lose some of your mystery' ... she seemed to take this but did not respond directly ....

Another day as the weather became warmer ... she was complaining about the sunshine and having to carry her heavy leather coat ... and I suggested again rather sharply that perhaps it was time to carry a lighter one .... To this she gave a girlish, 'Oooh no! It's my security blanket ... how can I do without it?' ... but she'd never have been able to laugh at herself like that in the early days ....

Soon after these sessions of ... what my supervisor had called negative therapeutic reaction had occurred ... in the later period of work ... she started work on resuming normal shopping expeditions ... to places further away from home that required the use of public transport .... She also made contact with her former boyfriend and went walking in the park with him ... and said she'd decided he was a true friend ....

Although her life will continue to be stressful, she now has much more freedom and has broken out of the vicious circle that kept her tied to home and fearful .... If we can end this work carefully she may feel able to seek more long term help in the future or to return here at a later date to carry our work together forward .... And in any event I'll be able to transfer her to the intermittent service (Service D) for a tailing-off period of up to a year after our fortnightly sessions have finished ....

## IN CONCLUSION ...

### Containment

- The form of containment offered was transformative.
- The GP had discussed with the patient other forms of containment, through drug treatment, but the patient chose brief weekly counselling.

### Outcomes

- Good. The patient met her own targets: to go out every day; to identify a true friend; to modify her relationship with her family inside herself.
- From the point of view of future prevention, the GP, counsellor and patient are all satisfied that the psychiatric services (outpatients, community mental health team, drugs, hospital) will not now be needed.
- The patient can now travel on public transport.
- The patient has recently been able to manage a rigorous review of her case at the benefits office, truthfully and with dignity, and hopes to be given support for training as a librarian.
- Several regressions have occurred and have been understood.
- The patient can have continuing help from the intermittent service (D) if she wants it, after her sessions finish.

## Multi-professional team

- GP and counsellor worked well together, using the exchange of records system after each appointment, but met only twice.
- Complementary therapy was not indicated for this patient, given her serious problems with revealing her body to anyone; massage therapy and/or homeopathy may be relevant at a later stage.
- The patient, for obvious reasons, preferred to have her help on site at the practice and did not want help from any other services.
- Reception staff, an important part of the overall team, were avoided and within the practice seemed to represent the officialdom of which the patient was so frightened: an issue for further work

## Postmodernism

- Global city: experienced by the patient as too fast, too big, too complex and overwhelming.
- Complexification: before her counselling, the prospect of going to other services for help, of having to negotiate legitimate but complex benefits at home or in the office, and of having to cope with the underground, were all too difficult for this patient.
- Impact of Technology: the patient's work as a secretary at home was facilitated; also, she was identified as a long term claimant of benefits at a time of benefit policy change, and could no longer hide away; subsequently her progress will be tracked.
- Commodification: the future cost to the NHS and other welfare services of patients with this kind of psychological problem was a factor in extending counselling at the practice beyond the usual limit.
- Superficial language games: the patient's dream moved the dialogue away from surface clichés about 'letting go' or 'leaving' into a deeper level, where internal emotional links were discovered between her present life, her family relationships in the past, and the sense of a future ending with the counsellor.

# PART 4

# The global city

# 15

# Inner world and inner city

*Marilyn Pietroni*

The truth, actually, is less romantic. Certain forms of consensus are so essential to community life that they re-establish themselves despite every attempt to shake them.

Umberto Eco, *Reports from the global village: travels in hyper-reality*

Change of heart is the most basic. Without stronger moral voices, public authorities are overburdened and markets don't work. Without moral commitments, people act without any consideration for one another. In recent years too many of us have been reluctant to lay moral claims on one another. It is a mistaken notion that because we desire to be free from governmental controls we should also be free from responsibilities to the commons, indifferent to the community.

Amitai Etzioni, *The spirit of community*

Life in the inner city can be a struggle for human connection, a struggle for a sense of belonging to some kind of community. For some, the health centre actually becomes that community, a kind of safe haven in which they relate to the receptionists, the GPs, the practice or district nurses, the volunteers and several members of the wider team. They send cards at Christmas or Hannukah or Diwali and bring small gifts into the practice, as they would to the family from which many are alienated or which many lack. For others, it is but one stopping off point in a network of fragmented but necessary connections that keep them afloat, as they veer between the NHS and private practice or between cooperation and conflict with different members of the health centre team. For others still, it is a rarely visited port in an unforeseen storm as they are struck by events: a serious illness, an accident, a bereavement, unemployment. We have given brief examples of these smaller pieces of work in the early chapters.

As inner city counsellors we have tried to show how, even in the fragmented and bitty world of general practice, the 'still points' of mutual human communication, however brief or transitory, should not be undervalued and can endure. Sometimes that communication merely helps someone to get through a difficult time, and may be more important for its process of human contact than its content; an example might be The Fractured Widow in Chapter 13. For others, like the Refugee Artist (Chapter 9) and the Torture Victim (Chapter 11), it is a necessary raft to hang on to over time, without which they might go under.

The majority of patients who come to us as counsellors, however, find it is a chance to do a piece of significant work that helps them to find a new direction and to go on growing and thinking about who they are and how they can actively shape their lives; examples here would be the young woman in Chapter 14, the older woman in Chapter 10, who psychically woke up to discover that she was in the winter of her life and had a lot of work to prepare herself for what was ahead, or the schoolgirl in Chapter 12, adjusting to life away from home.

Individual patients, the multi-professional team and the inter-agency network all struggle with the risks of fragmentation on the one hand and a drive for coherence on the other. Neither are necessarily productive in and of themselves, either for the professionals or for the patients; fragmentation can turn into mindless chaos, and coherence too easily flips over into a defensive order that serves the professionals' need for clarity, but not the patient's need for a combination of flexibility with limits. The tensions in inter-professional and inter-agency collaboration, between tolerating muddle, uncertainty and contradiction on the one hand, and seeking clarity and a common-enough language and protocols for practice on the other, are vital tensions; vital that is in the sense of showing signs of life. We will never and should never be without them, as Professor Carl Menninger said passionately at a conference on stress in Louisville in 1979, reflecting on his book *The Vital Balance* (Menninger, Mayman & Pruser 1963). He wished in his later life that he had called it *The Vital Imbalance*, because with imbalance there was always movement, and movement or stress was a sign of life; it needed harnessing but not too much.

That tension between order and chaos has naturally been with us in the writing of this book. We were often caught between a logical exposition of our work and the living reality of its unevenness, created not only by our own fluctuating human capacities but also by the extremes and ordinariness of the problems that patients bring to us. We have erred, perhaps inevitably, on the side of unevenness, because our reflective practice approach has taken the text much closer to our patients, our colleagues and ourselves than a more reasoned exposition would have allowed. As stated in Chapter 6, we have also sought to fill a gap in the literature by describing, warts and all, what actually happens in inner city counselling in one general practice: what we, and those around us in the primary care network, actually think, say and do. The sample of work described here has therefore not been selected on the basis of successful outcome, but in order to put in the public domain a typical slice of our experience.

Donald Schön, in his reflective practice laboratories, always pushed for the contradictions and the unexpected in practice examples brought to him for scrutiny. Michael and Enid Balint did the same with GPs bringing examples of general practice consultations to a 'Balint Group'. A 'harmonious interpenetrating mix-up' was how Michael Balint (1968) described the effort towards communication between two people, bonded in an intimate therapeutic endeavour but with a backdrop of sometimes more and sometimes less helpful theoretical frameworks and practice conventions. If we have conveyed something of that experience, then we will have sufficiently communicated what it is like to be counselling in the inner city at Marylebone Health Centre.

# Abbreviations and definitions

| | |
|---|---|
| A and E | Accident and Emergency |
| BAC | British Association for Counselling |
| BACCMS | British Association for Counselling: Counselling in Medical Settings Section |
| BAP | British Association of Psychotherapists |
| BCP | British Confederation of Psychotherapists |
| BPS | British Psychological Society |
| CAT | Cognitive Analytic Therapy |
| CBT | Cognitive Behavioural Therapy |
| CCCPH | Centre for Community Care and Primary Health, University of Westminster |
| CHI or CHIMP | Commission for Health Improvement |
| CMHT | Community Mental Health Team |
| CMS | Counselling in Medical Settings Section of BAC |
| CORE | Clinical Outcomes in Routine Evaluation (University of Leeds) |
| CPC | The Association of Counsellors in Primary Care |
| CPCT | Counselling in Primary Care Trust |
| CPR | Care Planning Review Meeting |
| DNA | Did not attend (of a patient) |
| FHSA | Family Health Services Authority |
| HA | Health Authority |
| HAZ | Health Action Zone |
| HIP | Health Improvement Plans |
| Inter-agency | Different agencies (social services, community health trusts, general practice, etc.) working collaboratively |

|  | with active awareness, understanding and use of their different agency policies and tasks |
|---|---|
| Inter-professional | Different professions working collaboratively with an active awareness, understanding and use of professional differences |
| Jarman Index | Underprivileged Area Score (developed by Dr Brian Jarman) |
| LATS | London Academic Training Scheme |
| LIZEI | London Implementation Zone Educational Initiative |
| MCT | Marylebone Centre Trust (Charity associated with Marylebone Health Centre) |
| MHC | Marylebone Health Centre |
| Multi-agency | Different agencies working together in parallel compartments on the same project without active, collaborative use of their differences |
| Multi-professional | Different professions working in parallel compartments without active collaboration or a team comprised of different professions |
| NCVQ | National Council for Vocational Qualifications |
| Network | Different agencies or professions who sometimes work together on specific cases or time-limited projects |
| NHSE | National Health Service Executive ('Leeds') |
| NICE | National Institute of Clinical Excellence |
| NVQ | National Vocational Qualification |
| PCG | Primary Care Group |
| PCT | Primary Care Team |
| PHCT | Primary Health Care Team |
| RCGP | Royal College of General Practitioners |
| RCP | Royal College of Psychiatrists |
| RCT | Randomized Control Trial |
| Team | A team of professionals who routinely work together over time on shared cases and enduring projects |

| UKCP | United Kingdom Council for Psychotherapy |
| UPA Score | Underprivileged Area Score (Jarman index) |
| UW or UoW | University of Westminster |
| WPF | Westminster Pastoral Foundation |

# References

Access to Health Records Act 1990 Stationery Office, London

Aldridge D, Pietroni P 1996 Research trials in general practice: towards a focus on clinical practice. In: Pietroni P, Pietroni C (eds) Innovation in community care and primary health: the Marylebone experiment. Churchill Livingstone, New York, pp. 168–72

Anderson S, Hasler J 1979 Counselling in general practice. Journal of the Royal College of General Practitioners 29:352–6

Argyris C, Schön DA 1974 Theory and practice: increasing professional effectiveness. Jossey Bass, San Francisco

Argyris C, Schön D 1978 Organisational learning: a theory of action perspective. Addison-Wesley, Reading, Ma

Atkins S, Murphy K 1993 Reflection: a review of the literature. Journal of Advanced Nursing 18:1188–1192

BAC 1993 Guidelines for the employment of counsellors in general practice. BAC, Rugby

BAC Research Network 1998 List of members. BAC, Rugby

Balint E 1973 The 'flash' technique: its freedom and its discipline. In: Balint E, Norell JS Six minutes for the patient: interactions in general practice consultations. Tavistock, London, pp. 19–32

Balint E, Norell JS (eds) 1973 Six minutes for the patient: interactions in general practice consultations. Tavistock, London

Balint E, Courtenay M, Elder A, Hull S, Julian P 1993 The doctor, the patient and the group: Balint revisited. Routledge, London

Balint M 1964 The doctor, his patient and the illness, 2nd edn. Pitman, London

Balint M 1968 The basic fault: therapeutic aspects of regression. Tavistock, London

Ball V 1993 Guidelines for the employment of counsellors in general practice. BAC, Rugby

Berger J 1989 Once in Europa. Granta, Cambridge

Bion W 1959 Attacks on linking. International Journal of Psychoanalysis 30:308–315

Bion W 1962 A theory of thinking. International Journal of Psycho-Analysis 33:306–310

Bion W 1965 Transformations. Heinemann, London

Bion W 1970 Attention and interpretation. Tavistock, London

Bond T 1995 The nature and outcomes of counselling. In: Keithley J & Marsh G (eds) Counselling in primary health care. Oxford University Press, pp. 3–26

Booth H, Goodwin I, Newnes C, Dawson O 1997 Process and outcome of counselling in general practice. Clinical Psychology Forum 101:32–40

Bor R 1987 Establishing, managing and evaluating counselling services. Cassell, London

Boud D, Keogh R, Walker D 1985 Reflection: turning experience into learning. Kegan Page, London

Box S, Copley B, Magagna J, Moustaki E 1981 Psychotherapy with families: an analytic approach. Routledge, London

Brook A, Temperley J 1976 The contribution of a psychotherapist to general practice. Journal of the Royal College of General Practitioners 26:86–94

Bruggen P, Byng-Hall J, Pitt-Aitken T 1973 The reason for admission as the focus of work in an inpatient adolescent unit. British Journal of Psychiatry 122:319–329

Burton M 1995 Evaluating the work of counsellors in general practice. In: Supplement 2. CPCT, Staines

Burton M 1998 Psychotherapy, counselling and primary health care: assessment for brief and longer term treatment. John Wiley, London

Burton M, Henderson P, Curtis Jenkins G 1998 Primary care counsellors' experiences of supervision. Counselling 9(2):122–133

Caplan G 1964 Principles of preventive psychiatry. Tavistock, London, pp. 81–88

Chase D, Davies P 1991 The calculation of a practice underprivileged area (UPA) score. In: Pietroni P, Pietroni C (eds) 1996 Innovation in community care and primary health: the Marylebone experiment. Churchill Livingstone, New York, pp. 47–52

CORE System Group 1998 CORE system (information management) handbook. CORE System Group, Leeds

Corney R 1993 Studies of the effectiveness of counselling in general practice. In Corney R, Jenkins R (eds) Counselling in general practice. Routledge, London

Corney R 1996 Links between mental health professionals and general practices in England and Wales: the impact of GP fundholding. British Journal of General Practice 46:221–4

Corney R 1997 Counselling in the medical context. In: Palmer S, McMahon G (eds) Handbook of counselling, 2nd edn. Routledge, London, pp. 161–75

Corney R 1999 Evaluating clinical counselling in primary care. In: Lees J (ed) Clinical counselling in general practice. Routledge, London

Corney R, Jenkins R (eds) 1993 Counselling in general practice. Routledge, London

Curtis Jenkins G 1992 Reasons for failure of counselling in general practice. CPCT, Staines

Curtis Jenkins G 1995a The complete guide to counselling in general practice. Pulse 3 (June):65–73

Curtis Jenkins G 1995b Does counselling work? Update (1 April):413–414

Curtis Jenkins G 1996 A guide to counselling in general practice. In: Supplement 2. CPCT, Staines

Curtis Jenkins G 1997 Setting the scene: supervision of counsellors in general practice, a four-fold model. In: Supervision: Supplement 3. CPCT, Staines

Curtis Jenkins G 1998a Reflections on general practice counselling and the need for organisation and regulation. Counselling in Primary Care conference proceedings. Counselling in Primary Care Today and Tomorrow: 98–106. CMS/CPCT/Mole Conferences, London

Curtis Jenkins G 1998b Counsellors in general practice. Community Mental Health Today (forthcoming)

Dammers J, Wiener J 1995 The theory and practice of counselling in the primary health care team. In: Keithley J, Marsh G (eds) Counselling in primary health care. Oxford University Press, Oxford pp. 27–56

Davidson L, Curtis Jenkins G, Mellor-Clark J 1997 Clinical effectiveness and primary care counselling: guidance for purchasers and providers. Unpublished paper, National Network of Counselling in Primary Care

Department of Health 1987 White Paper: Promoting better health. HMSO, London

Department of Health 1989 White Paper: Working for patients. HMSO, London

Department of Health 1990 NHS and Community Care Act. HMSO, London

Department of Health 1991a White Paper: The health of the nation. HMSO, London

Department of Health 1991b The Patient's Charter. HMSO, London

Department of Health 1996a White Paper: Choice and opportunity. HMSO, London

Department of Health 1996b White Paper: A service with ambition. HMSO, London

Department of Health 1996c White Paper: Delivering the future. HMSO, London

Department of Health 1997 White Paper: The new NHS: modern – dependable. HMSO, London

Department of Health 1998a Green Paper: Our healthier nation. HMSO, London

Department of Health 1998b Action Paper: Modernizing health and social services. HMSO, London

Dowrick C 1992 Improving mental health through primary care. British Journal of General Practice 42:382–6

East P 1995 Counselling in medical settings. Open University Press, Buckingham

Eco U 1986 Reports from the global village: travels in hyper-reality. Picador, London

Elder A, Samuel O (eds) 1987 While I'm here, Doctor: a study of the doctor-patient relationship. Tavistock, London

Eliot TS 1944 The four-quartets: Burnt Norton. Faber and Faber, London, pp. 15–16

Elton Wilson J 1996 Time-conscious psychological therapy. Routledge, London

Eraut M 1995 Schön shock: a case for reframing reflection-in-action? Teachers and teaching: theory and practice 1(1):9–22

Etzioni A 1993 The spirit of community. Fontana, London, p. 247

Feltham C 1997 Time-limited counselling. Sage, London

Fernando S 1995 Social realities and mental health. In: Fernando S (ed.) Mental health in a multi-ethnic society. Routledge, London

Firth M, Rowlands C M 1997 Psychiatric social work in primary care: a pilot scheme in one inner city practice. Journal of Interprofessional Care XI(3)

Freud S 1914 Remembering, repeating and working through. In: Further recommendations on the technique of psychoanalysis II. SE XII:157–166. Hogarth, London

Freud S 1923 The ego and the id. SE XIX:3–66. Hogarth, London

Garret B 1990 Creating the learning organization: a guide to leadership, learning and development. Director Books, Cambridge

Ginzburg N 1986 Family sayings. Paladin, London

Graham M 1995 The counsellor's perspective. In: Keithley J, Marsh G (eds) Counselling in primary health care, Oxford University Press, Oxford

Gustafson J P 1986 The complex secret of brief psychotherapy. Jason Aronson, Northvale, NJ

Gustafson J P 1995a Brief versus long psychotherapy: when, why and how. Jason Aronson, Northvale, NJ

Gustafson J P 1995b The dilemmas of brief psychotherapy. Plenum, New York

Hamilton Noël-Paton M 1984 War widow. In: Chaos of the night. Virago, London

Harris C 1987 Let's do away with counselling. In: Medical annual: the yearbook of general practice. Wright, Bristol

Harris M 1994 Magic in the surgery: counselling and the NHS. Social Affairs Unit, London

Hemmings A 1996 Counselling in primary care: is it as effective as routine treatment? 5th St George's Counselling in Primary Care Conference: The future: professional registration, effectiveness and new ways of working. St George's Conference Unit, London: 30–40

Henderson P 1993 Postgraduate diploma in counselling in primary health care. CPCT, Staines

Hicks R 1994 Report of counselling in KCW general practices. Kensington, Chelsea and Westminster Commissioning Agency, London

Hinshelwood R 1991 A dictionary of Kleinian thought. Free Association Books, London

Hoag L 1992 Psychotherapy in the GP surgery: considerations of the frame. British Journal of Psychotherapy 8:417–429

Hoggett P 1992 Partisans in an uncertain world: the psychoanalysis of engagement. Free Association Books, London

Horney K 1936 The problem of negative therapeutic reaction. Psychoanalytic Quarterly 5:29–44

House R 1997 The dynamics of professionalism: a personal view of counselling research. Counselling (August) 8(3):200–204

Hughes P 1996 Learning to integrate: facts and feelings in medical education. 2nd Working Across Cultures conference proceedings: 15–24. St George's Mental Health Library, Conference Series 1996, London

Huntington J 1993 From FPC to FHSA to … health commission? British Medical Journal 306:33–36

Hurd J, Rowland N 1991 Counselling in general practice: a guide for counsellors, 2nd edn. BAC, Rugby

Irving J, Heath V 1989 Counselling in general practice: a guide for general practitioners, 2nd edn. BAC, Rugby

Jameson F 1991 Postmodernism or the cultural logic of late capitalism. Verso, London

Jarman B 1983 Identification of underprivileged areas. British Medical Journal 286:1705–1709

Jarman B 1984 Underprivileged areas: validation and distribution of scores. British Medical Journal 290:1714–1716

Jarman B 1988 Primary care. Heinemann, London

Jenkins R, Shepherd M 1983 Mental illness and general practice. In: Bean P (ed) Mental illness: changes and trends. John Wiley, London, ch 15, pp. 403–409

Jones H, Murphy A, Neaman G, Tollemache R, Vasserman D 1994 Psychotherapy and counselling in a GP practice: making use of the setting. British Journal of Psychotherapy 10(4):543–551

Keithley J 1995 Counselling in primary care. Oxford University Press, Oxford

Keithley J, Marsh G (eds) 1995 Counselling in primary health care. Oxford University Press, Oxford

Klein M 1946 Notes on some schizoid mechanisms. International Journal of Psychoanalysis 27:99–110

Klein R 1998 Clinical depression. Guardian, Society section, 29 April

Kolb D 1984 Experiental learning. Prentice-Hall, Englewood Cliffs, NJ

Kristeva J 1984 In conversation with Rosalind Coward. In: Desire, ICA Documents 22–27. ICA, London

Laplanche J, Pontalis J-B 1980 The language of psychoanalysis. Hogarth Press and Institute of Psychoanalysis, London

Launer J 1994 Psychotherapy in the general practice surgery: working with and without a secure therapeutic frame. British Journal of Psychotherapy 11(1):120–126

Leathard A 1996 Going interprofessional. Routledge, London

Lees J 1997 An approach to counselling in GP surgeries. Psychodynamic Counselling 3(1):33–48

Lees J (ed) 1999 Clinical counselling in general practice. Routledge, London

Lowell A 1992 Circumstance. In: Imagist poetry. Penguin, p. 89

Lyotard J-F 1984 The postmodern condition: a report on knowledge. Manchester University Press, Manchester

Mackenzie B 1996 The enemy within: an exploration of the concept of boundaries in a GP surgery. Psychodynamic Counselling 2(3)

McLeod J 1988 The work of counsellors in general practice. Occasional Paper 37, Royal College of General Practitioners, London

Malan D H 1963 A study of brief psychotherapy. Tavistock, London

Malan D H 1976a The frontier of brief psychotherapy: an example of the convergence of research and clinical practice 2nd edn. Plenum, New York

Malan D H 1976b Toward the validation of dynamic psychotherapy. Plenum, New York

Malan D H 1979 Individual psychotherapy and the science of psychodynamics. Butterworth, London

Malan D H, Osimo F 1992 Psychodynamics, training and outcome in brief psychotherapy. Butterworth-Heinemann, Oxford

Mann A 1993 The need for counselling: the extent of psychiatric and psychosocial disorders in primary care – a review of the epidemiological research findings. In: Corney R, Jenkins R (eds) Counselling in general practice. Routledge, London, pp. 7–16

Mann J 1973 Time-limited psychotherapy. Harvard University Press, Cambridge, Ma.

Marsh G N 1993 The counsellor as part of the general practice team. In: Corney R, Jenkins R (eds) Counselling in general practice. Routledge, London, pp. 67–74

Marsh G N, Barr J 1975 Marriage guidance counselling in a group practice. Journal of the Royal College of General Practitioners 25:73–75

Martin E, Mitchell H 1983 A counsellor in general practice: a one year survey. Journal of the Royal College of General Practitioners 33:366–367

Marylebone Health Centre 1992–1998 Annual audit. Marylebone Health Centre, London

Maynard A 1995 Introduction. In: Tolley K, Rowland N Evaluating the cost-effectiveness of counselling in health care. Routledge, London

Mellor-Clark J 1998 CORE system update. Counselling in Practice 2(3):10

Meltzer D 1978 Container and contained: the prototype of learning. The Kleinian development Part III: The clinical significance of the work of Bion. Clunie, Perthshire

Menninger C, Mayman M, Pruser P 1963 The vital balance: the life process in mental health and illness. Viking, New York

Menzies Lyth I 1988 Containing anxiety in institutions: selected essays. Free Association Books, London

Mezirow J 1981 A critical theory of adult learning and education. Adult Education 32(1):3–24

Mohamed C, Smith R 1997 Race in the therapy relationship. In: Lawrence M, Maguire M (eds) Psychotherapy with women: feminist perspectives. Macmillan, London, pp. 134–159

Molnos A 1995 A question of time. Karnac Books, London

Moustaki E 1981 Glossary: a discussion and application of terms. In: Box S, Copley B, Magagna J, Moustaki E Psychotherapy with families: an analytic approach. Routledge, London

NHS Centre for Reviews and Dissemination 1997 Mental health promotion in high risk groups. Effective Health Care 3(3)

Noonan E 1983 Counselling young people. Methuen, London

North and South Derbyshire Health Authorities 1993 Guidelines and protocols for the employment of counsellors in general practice, 3rd edn.

Parry G 1995 Bambi fights back: psychotherapy research and service improvement. Changes 13:154–167.

Parry G 1997 Psychotherapy services in the English National Health Service. In: Miller N E, Magruder K (eds) The cost-effectiveness of psychotherapy: a guide for practitioners, researchers and policymakers. Wiley, New York

Parton N 1994 'The problematics of government' (post)modernity and social work. British Journal of Social Work 24:9–32

Pietroni M 1993 Validation document: MA in Community and Primary Health Care: Towards reflective practice. University of Westminster, London

Pietroni M 1995 The nature and aims of professional education for social workers: a postmodern perspective. In: Yelloly M, Henkel M (eds) Learning and teaching in social work: towards reflective practice. Jessica Kingsley, London and Bristol

Pietroni M 1999 The postmodern context of counselling in general practice: the impact of the NHS and Community Care Act 1990. In: Lees J (ed) Clinical counselling in general practice. Routledge, London

Pietroni P 1996a Introduction. In: Pietroni P, Pietroni C (eds) Innovation in community care and primary health the Marylebone experiment. Churchill Livingstone, Edinburgh, pp. xvii–xix

Pietroni P 1996b Towards reflective practice: the languages of health and social care. In: Pietroni P, Pietroni C (eds) Innovation in community care and primary health: the Marylebone experiment. Churchill Livingstone, Edinburgh, pp. 32–41

Pietroni P 1996c Issues in research and methodology. In: Pietroni P, Pietroni C (eds) Innovation in community care and primary health: the Marylebone experiment. Churchill Livingstone, Edinburgh, pp. 165–167

Pietroni P, d'Uray Ura S 1994 Informal complaints procedures in general practice – a one year audit. British Medical Journal 308:1546–1549.

Pietroni P, Pietroni C (eds) 1996 Innovation in community care and primary health: the Marylebone experiment. Churchill Livingstone, Edinburgh

Rain L 1997 Counselling in primary care: a guide to good practice. MIND Counselling in Primary Care Project, Leeds

Richards B 1994 Disciplines of delight. Free Association Books, London

Roberts J 1997 Where ethical codes meet with managerial control: the business culture and its effects on the theory and practice of psychodynamic counselling – or some thoughts on hiring and firing. Psychodynamic Counselling 3(1):83–88

Rosenfeld H 1952 Notes on the analysis of the super-ego conflict in an acute catatonic schizophrenic. International Journal of Psycho-Analysis 33:111–131

Roth A, Fonagy P 1996 What works for whom? A critical review of psychotherapy research. Guilford Press, New York and London

Rowland N, Irving J 1984 Towards a rationalization of counselling in general practice. Journal of the Royal College of General Practitioners 34:685–687

Rowland N, Irving J, Maynard A 1989 Can general practitioners counsel? Journal of the Royal College of General Practitioners 39:118–120

Rustin M 1991 The good society and the inner world: psychoanalysis, politics and culture. Verso, London

Ryle A 1990 Cognitive analytic therapy: active participation in change – a new integration in brief psychotherapy. John Wiley, Chichester

Saïd E 1993 Culture and imperialism. Chatto and Windus, London

Samskrti and Veda 1976 Hatha yoga manual. Himalayan Institute, Honesdale, Pennsylvania

Sanders K 1986 A matter of interest: notes of a psycho-analyst in general practice. Clunie Press, Perthshire

Schön D A 1963 The displacement of concepts: public and private learning in a changing society. Tavistock, London

Schön D A 1970 The loss of the stable state. Reith Lecture, The Listener (19 November) 84 (2173:685–688)

Schön D A 1971 Beyond the stable state. Temple Smith, London

Schön D A 1987a The reflective practitioner: how professionals think in action. Jossey Bass, San Francisco

Schön D A 1987b Educating the reflective practitioner. Jossey Bass, San Francisco

Schön D A 1991 The reflective practitioner, 2nd edn. Jossey Bass, San Francisco

Schön D A 1992 The crisis of professional knowledge and the pursuit of an epistemology of practice. Journal of Interprofessional Care 6(1):49–63

Sedgwick-Taylor A 1996 The Gloucester experience: a practical example of how a counsellor can make the difference. 5th St George's Counselling in Primary Care Conference. The future: professional registration, effectiveness and new ways of working: 41–77. St George's Conference Unit, London

Sheldon M (ed) 1992 Counselling in general practice. Royal College of General Practitioners Clinical Series, Exeter

Sher M 1992 Dynamic teamwork within general medical practice. Proceedings from Counselling in Primary Care Conference, British Association of Psychiatry

Sibbald B 1998 Foreword. In: Wiener J, Sher M 1998 Counselling and psychotherapy in primary health care: a psychodynamic approach. Macmillan, London, p. xiv

Sibbald B, Addington Hall J, Brenneman D, Freeling P 1993 Counsellors in English and Welsh general practices: their nature and distribution. British Medical Journal 306:29–33

Sibbald B, Addington Hall J, Brenneman D, Freeling P 1996a The role of counsellors in general practice: a qualitative study. Occasional Paper 74, Royal College of General Practitioners, London

Sibbald B, Elder A, Jenkins R, Wiener J, Higgs R 1996b Primary care and psychotherapy. In: Future directions of psychotherapy in the NHS: adaptation or extinction? Conference proceedings. Psychoanalytic Psychotherapy 10(Supplement): 57–120

Sibbald B, Addington Hall J, Brenneman D et al 1996c Investigation of whether on-site general practice counsellors have an impact on psychotropic drug prescribing rates and costs. British Journal of General Practice 46:63–67

Sifneos P E 1972 Short-term psychotherapy and emotional crisis. Harvard University Press, Cambridge, Ma

Smith P 1992 The emotional labour of nursing. Macmillan, Basingstoke

Spratley J, Pietroni M 1994 Creative collaboration: interprofessional learning priorities in primary health and community care. Report of a project undertaken by Marylebone Centre Trust on behalf of CCETSW. Marylebone Centre Trust, London

Stern D 1985 The interpersonal world of the infant: a view from psychoanalysis and development psychology. Basic Books, New York

Summerfield D 1996 Understanding experiences: war and refugeeism. 25th Annual Training Event and Conference, Association for Student Counselling / Forum Européen de l'orientation académique: 72–77. BAC, Rugby

Symington J, Symington N 1996 The clinical thinking of Wilfrid Bion. Routledge, London

Terry P 1997 Counselling the elderly and their carers. Macmillan, London

Tolley K, Rowland N 1995 Evaluating the cost-effectiveness of counselling in health care. Routledge, London

Tomlinson D 1992 Report of the enquiry into London's health service. HMSO, London

Toulmin S 1990 Cosmopolis. University of Chicago Press, Chicago

Ward I 1997 The presentation of case material in clinical discourse. Freud Museum, London

Waydenfeld D, Waydenfeld S W 1980 Counselling in general practice. Journal of the Royal College of General Practitioners 30:671–677

Webber V, Davies P, Pietroni P 1996 Counselling in an inner city general practice: analysis of its use and uptake. In: Pietroni P, Pietroni C (eds) Innovation in community care and primary health: the Marylebone experiment. Churchill Livingstone, Edinburgh, pp. 132–137

Widgery D 1991 Some lives. Sinclair-Stevenson, London

Wiener J 1996 Primary care and psychotherapy. In: Future directions of psychotherapy within the NHS: adaptation or extinction? Conference proceedings. Psychoanalytic Psychotherapy 10 (Supplement)

Wiener J, Sher M 1998 Counselling and psychotherapy in primary health care: a psychodynamic approach. Macmillan, London

Wing J, Curtis R, Beever A 1996 HoNOS: Health of the Nation Outcome Scores: brief report. Royal College of Psychiatrists, College Research Unit, London

Winnicott D W 1971 The good enough. In: Playing and reality. Tavistock, London

Wylde K L 1981 Counselling in general practice: a review. Journal of Guidance and Counselling 9

# Index